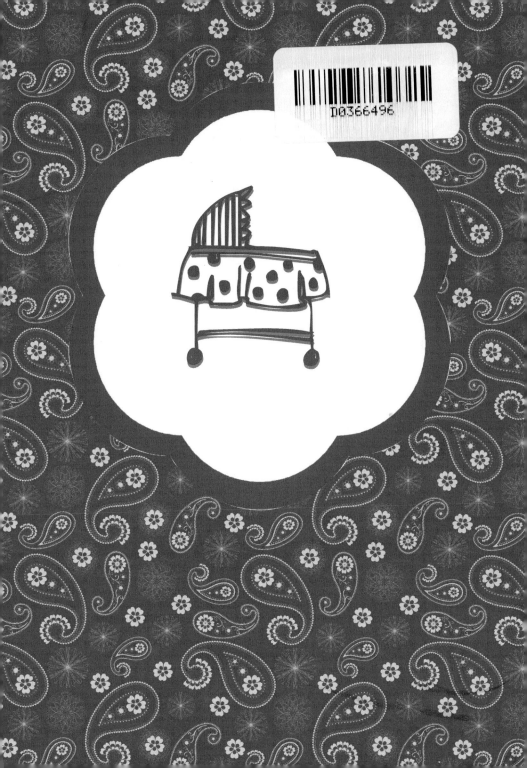

THE UNEXPECTED WHEN YOU'RE EXPECTING

(a parody)

The UNEXPECTED WHEN YOU'RE EXPECTING

CLEAR, COMPREHENSIVE, MONTH-BY-MONTH DREAD

MARY K. MOORE

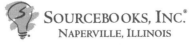

SOURCEBOOKS, INC.®
NAPERVILLE, ILLINOIS

Published by Sourcebooks, Inc.
P.O. Box 4410, Naperville, Illinois 60567–4410
(630) 961–3900
Fax: (630) 961–2168
www.sourcebooks.com

Library of Congress Cataloging-in-Publication Data

Moore, Mary K.
  The unexpected when you're expecting : the pregnancy guide that will make you
rue the night of conception / Mary K. Moore.
       p. cm.
  1. Pregnancy—Humor. I. Title.
  PN6231.P68M66 2008
  818'.602—dc22
                              2008015870

Printed and bound in the United States of America.
POD 10 9 8 7 6 5 4 3

For T.J. and Scarlett, who are in on the joke.

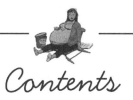

Contents

THE UNEXPECTED WHEN YOU'RE EXPECTING

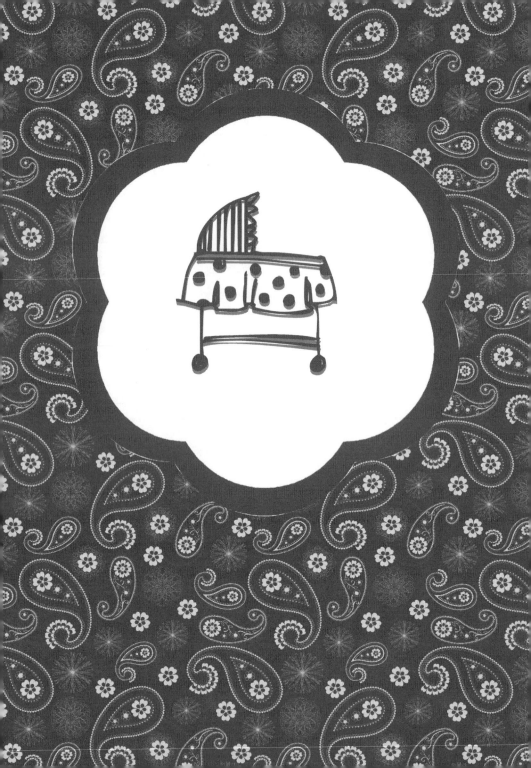

CHAPTER 1

Preggers:
Yes or No?

You think you might be pregnant. Immediately, you have visions of your glowing, radiant body blossoming into motherhood (except, of course, your arms, legs, butt, and face.) You'll buy a few empire-waist dresses, temporarily trade your heels for cute flats, and try to get used to being the center of attention.

Think again. Welcome to invasion of the body snatchers. Only this time, it's an inside job. Congratulations. You're pregnant.*

Reminder:

If you're Caucasian, say goodbye to those pink nipples, sweetie. You're headed to brown town.

WHAT YOU MAY BE FREAKED OUT ABOUT

"The pregnancy tests and my ob-gyn say no, but I just know that they're wrong. Could the doctor be messing with my head or dipping the wrong woman's urine?"

*Oh, just so you know, forty weeks isn't nine months—it's ten. Liars!

You're delusional. Snap out of it. You can always have a vagina like a garage later. Go have a drink and a cigarette—even if you're not a smoker—for all those women out there for whom fun and vices will soon be a bitter, distant memory.

Knowing for Sure: Test Time

Welcome to the section of the pharmacy you didn't know existed. Move away from the lubes and products with silhouetted lovers and go toward the cooing infants. This is because there is no truth in advertising. If there were, you'd be looking for the image of the woman slapping her forehead or molesting a pint of ice cream. And get ready to piss on your hand. If you're normal, you'll have no idea about the trajectory of your own urine. If you're a marksman, it's probably because of some bizarre sorority pledging rite, which might be why you're here in the first place.

But first you must pick a predictor. You'll find everything from off-name brands (Wee & Weep) to commercial favorites (E.P.T. Early Pregnancy Test: "What if you could know the moment you became pregnant?" or its lesser-known companion, E.P.T.E.S.P.: "What if you could know if you'd become pregnant in the future?") The choices are limitless, unlike your clothing options in the months ahead.

The display results vary with each test. Thanks to nervous women glutting up the pharmaceutical company's 800-number in double-line denial, wise product engineers have devised tests that now say "pregnant" or "not pregnant." (The standard "positive" or "not positive," as it turns out, all depends on your perspective. Just ask a jubilant-then-immediately-devastated teen.)

The In-Office Verdict

Now it's starting to sink in. You know you're pregnant. You're at the clinic, for chrissake. A blood test is just going to tell the doctor what you already know—you're terribly absent-minded when you're horny.

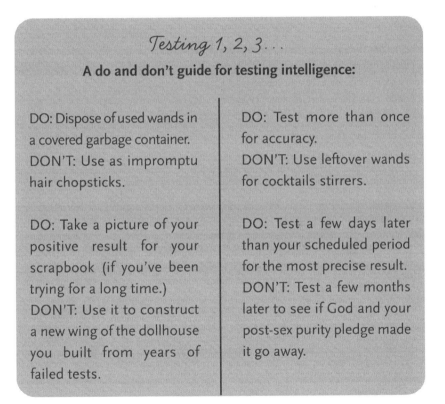

Testing 1, 2, 3...

A do and don't guide for testing intelligence:

DO: Dispose of used wands in a covered garbage container.
DON'T: Use as impromptu hair chopsticks.

DO: Take a picture of your positive result for your scrapbook (if you've been trying for a long time.)
DON'T: Use it to construct a new wing of the dollhouse you built from years of failed tests.

DO: Test more than once for accuracy.
DON'T: Use leftover wands for cocktails stirrers.

DO: Test a few days later than your scheduled period for the most precise result.
DON'T: Test a few months later to see if God and your post-sex purity pledge made it go away.

Let's Get Physical

This will be performed by either your ob-gyn or, if you're generally misguided, a midwife. You'll be asked to position yourself on the examining table or kitchen counter (see latter) with legs in stirrups. If given the choice, ask for a male physician. Then close your eyes and pretend you had a nice dinner together. Honestly, this is the last time in many months a man will look directly at your sugar walls without silently lamenting, *Do I have to?* Enjoy.

Of note, it is possible to experience all of the symptoms of pregnancy and not be pregnant at all. That's either called being crazy or dating a star NFL/NBA player.

Breaking the News...

Once you know for sure, it's time to share it with the person you now have by the balls. Here are some creative ways to make it official:

- Leave the positive test on the sink and scrawl on the bathroom mirror: "Meet me at Babies "R" Us with your wallet and a U-haul."
- Give him a sterling silver rattle with "I think it's yours" engraved on it.
- Have the waiter place a personalized message in a fortune cookie: "Confucius say a third of your paycheck is now mine."

CHAPTER 2

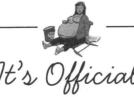

It's Official: Your Belly's in Charge

The blood tests are back, and the reality is starting to seep in. You may have a list of questions that are growing along with that little tadpole: how many weeks until I have to pay through the nose for ugly maternity outfits? Is there anything I can do to prevent the scrapbooking instinct from kicking in? These are all normal and natural concerns. Relax. The following information will be as easy to digest as the now-forbidden caffeine you used to down by the vat. Read on.

YOUR BODY AND, YOU KNOW, WHAT TO DO WITH IT

Eating for Two (Not Four or Five)

Hey there, sister. It's not just you taking whippets of spray cheese or hitting the crack pipe anymore. Baby has a vested interest in your intake and will soon be siphoning bodily fluids like a junior on prom night. That means you'll have to make sure your eating and drinking habits pass the prenatal muster. This may include eating more fruits and vegetables, drinking lots of water, and cutting back on toad-licking.

Chips, Ahoy!

"I eat tons of junk food. In fact my fingertips frequently have an orange, radioactive glow. How can I eat better now that I'm pregnant?"

First, it's important to be able to recognize when a food is bad for you. Although some choices are obvious (deep-fried Coke, intravenous Krispy Kreme) there are some choices that fly under the nutritional radar. Here are some telltale signs to help you decipher the good, the bad, and the delicious.

- Does it turn your teeth purple but isn't wine?
- Is the word "ranch" used, but a cow is not a part of the equation?
- Can it also be purchased at a state fair?
- Do you have to flatten yourself on the ground to reach it on a store shelf?

How to Keep Your Paws out of the Cookie Jar

It's easy to forget that everything you consume goes on baby's prenatal plate, especially when you've already peeled back that roll of cookie dough and gnawed six inches off. Seductive as he may be, the Pillsbury Dough Boy isn't going to be there to help you lug that hefty sugar bag you'll call your baby. But it's never too late to make the right choices to prevent an Orson Welles-ian offspring. (Well, that's not entirely true. The eighth or ninth month, or after the birth for example, would all be considered too late.) If you must keep off-limits foods in your house (say, for spouse's sweet tooth) make them as difficult to reach as possible. One solution is to set up a perilous pregnancy obstacle course between you and forbidden treats. (Mallomar moat?) That way, you'll have to weigh real consequences (ruptured spleen) over less concrete, caloric ones (Three-Cheese Doritos).

Not Looking Pregnant from Behind

Exercising while pregnant is a great way to keep pounds at bay and improve post-birth recovery. But know this: you're going to be a spectacle. Teetering on the treadmill, you can be assured the gym managers will view you as one big lumbering lawsuit. But don't give up on a daily dose of feeling the burn (outside of your constant UTIs). Staying in shape will not only strengthen you during the pregnancy, it will hasten your postpartum recovery, making you do-able again that much sooner. Of course, there is always too much of a good thing, and a mom who strives to be fit must know where to draw the line. Activities to avoid include:

- Ultimate fighting
- Alligator wrestling
- Bull running
- Flugtagging (if you don't know what it is, all the better)

For those who are new to the fitness arena but want to take on some safer prenatal activity, recommendations include:

- Competitive knitting

- Extreme bird watching
- All-out origami
- Marathon napping
- Super-sizing

Staying Healthy While Losing Sight of Your Feet...

As you enter the first trimester, you may be concerned about what does and doesn't affect the health of a newborn. This generally includes any negative intakes like alcohol, caffeine, or episodes of *Two and a Half Men*. That said, there are ways to put a halt to leftover habits from your pre-baby life. Here are some possible alternatives for those now-that-you're-pregnant no-nos.

Instead of: Smoking Try: Arson	Instead of: Hosting cocktails Try: Hosting a cockfight
Instead of: Slugging a cup of coffee Try: Snorting a Pixie Stick	Instead of: Avoiding physical activity Try: Avoiding the physically attractive

You may also be concerned about the appropriate range of exercise. Can I still play tennis? Race cars? Joust? Maybe your work requires unusual physical strain or exposes you to hazardous environments (carnie, television writer, personal assistant to a celebrity). If you have any reservations, just consult the doctor who already hates you. What's one more question in a litany of annoying inquiries?

BIRTHING OPTIONS: MULTIPLE WAYS TO WRECK YOUR TAIL

Hell in Your Own Bed

Never in history have women had so many choices when it comes to childbirth and never before have they made such piss-poor decisions. Leave it to a bunch of moms with too much time on their hands to see just how far they can go to make delivering a baby that much more life-threatening. None of these quilt-handlers would dream of removing a loose tooth with a wrench at home *sans* Novocain, but when it comes to removing *a human from a vagina*, Aunt Faye armed with salad tongs is just as good as "them there medical doctors." Keep that sewing needle close, Auntie. You'll need it to stitch up the gaping cavern that used to be a perineum. (Rename it "vaganus"?)

Birthing Centers: The Pinnacle of Granola Gestation

If you at least have enough sense not to endanger your life at home but not enough to stop buying expensive organic crap, then chances are, a birthing center is for you. Once inside, you'll be knocked down by the smell of ylang-ylang candles, which help mask the stench of looming death. Birthing centers are often touted for their peaceful environments, unburdened by such medical extras like fetal monitoring or professionals who can save lives. Call a Code Blue and at most, you might get some extra pillows and a cup of herbal tea—*stat!* No labor inducing here, my friend. Your resident midwife will make sure nature takes its course, so go ahead and quit your job and have your mail forwarded. So, what are the reasons women turn to birthing centers? Some women want to include family members—read *children*—to witness the birth in a relaxed environment. (Guess who's bringing the placenta to show-and-tell?) Other women love the at-home convenience. Centers often have in-room kitchens, comfy furniture, or sleeping quarters for their spouse and family. Or you could just ruin the sheets of your local Motel 6 for a third of the cost.

Alternative Birth: High on High Mortality

WATER BIRTH: BREATHING IS FOR LOSERS

You just brought yourself to the brink of death giving birth, so why not take baby along with you? Welcome to water birth, where granola moms cross the line from being mildly annoying to dangerously ignorant. Unless you coupled with a merman nine months back or did a tremendous amount of LSD, it's doubtful your baby will come equipped with a set of gills. Besides, if you're willing to breast-feed until they can independently order steak, why not give them the advantage of, uh, *air* in those first precious moments? Oh, and treat yourself to a swig of oxygen while you're at it.

SHHHHH

Thanks to those wacky and loveable Scientologists, Hollywood and the just plain-old indoctrinated are starting to buzz about silent births (albeit keeping the buzzing noise to an absolute minimum). Tom and Katie were reported to have practiced a silent birth, perhaps not unlike their night of conception. Specifically, in silent birth, the atmosphere and the birthing woman should be as quiet as possible during the entire labor. In fact, extensive research by L. Ron Hubbard, the father of Scientology, has shown that a disruptive environment during birth can affect a baby for a lifetime. And since he had a vagina and all, and had felt someone erupting from his personal Krakatoa, he probably knew, right? Take a note, L.: when it comes to telling a woman how to push out eight pounds, silence is golden.

Hospital Birth: Where Authority Meets Apathy

Sure, you probably won't die, but your spirit will. If you thought the conception was clinical, welcome to the shiny world of speculums, forceps, and condescension. Of course, there is some time for levity—specifically, when you present them with your birth plan. Nurses will pass it around the lounge and, between mouthfuls of Bundt cake, bray at how you wanted "mood music" and "mid-labor acupressure." *Hahahahahahahaha!*

At hospitals in bigger cities, your bed will likely be touching another's, allowing you to share the immediate postpartum journey with that of a stranger and her extended family. If you choose a private room, you might feel tempted to look for the hooker that must come inclusive with the $700 fee. Sadly, this is one screwing with no happy ending.

HOW TO MAKE YOUR DOCTOR WISH HE'D NEVER GONE TO MED SCHOOL

Do you consider yourself well-informed? Do you research the Internet for the latest obstetric advances to discuss with your ob-gyn? Do you always remember to log all symptoms throughout your early pregnancy journey for you and your physician to discuss? Well then chances are, your doctor secretly hates you and having to stare into your meddling vulva just makes her loathe you that much more. To ensure you don't make it into her dinner conversation about "the pregnant idiot I saw today," here are some guidelines for appropriate physician-patient etiquette.

Acceptable: Using the doctor's email to ask brief medical questions
Not Acceptable: Forwarding him anything with the subject line "ANGELS"

Acceptable: Asking how long she has practiced as an ob-gyn
Not Acceptable: Asking if she's had any celebrity cooch sightings

Acceptable: Being completely up-front about your medical history
Not Acceptable: Being completely up-front about the conception

Acceptable: Asking if they'll accept your insurance
Not Acceptable: Asking if they'll accept your savior

WHAT YOU MAY BE FREAKED OUT ABOUT
Piggy-Back Pregnancies

"Six weeks after my first child was born, I became pregnant again. Is 'birth chasing' going to impact my well-being or that of my baby?"

Listen,…Listen… Listen… No, I'm not repeating myself. That's the echo in your birth canal. Who's having sex a month and a half after having a baby? You should be tired to the bone and, frankly, too tired to bone. If not, chances are, you're neglecting your baby to CPS proportions. Need proof? When they said your baby needed shots, you offered your set from Cancun. You asked if Red Bull came in formula packets. Face it. You make Tara Reid look like Donna Reed. At least those two unlucky souls will have someone to cling to and commiserate with in the years of therapy ahead.

After You've Finally Given Away All Your First Baby's Clothes

"This is my second time to be pregnant, but it's been a few years since my last pregnancy. Just enough time for me to forget all the horrible stuff and do it all over again. What will be the same and what will be different this time around?"

Well, the mother will be the same. You'll also be using the same uterus as in your previous pregnancy. The wonder you experienced in the first pregnancy will also be the same: wondering how you're going to afford this second mouth, and if baby number two will save your faltering relationship. What will be different is that you'll have to explain to your first child that there is a sibling on the way. Here are some possible openers to help ease your firstborn into the role of big brother or sister:

- "It looks like you're going to have to really step up your game."
- "Remember that attractive man who cleaned our pool this summer?"
- "We both know that we've been growing apart for some time..."
- "I think too much attention has made you a flaming narcissist."

Jealous Friends High-Five!

"I'm starting my pregnancy on the thin side—thinner than I've ever been in my life. Now I've gone and ruined it by getting pregnant. Is my enviable, soon-to-be-gone waif bod going to affect my baby's growth and development?"

No, but you'll look hot a lot longer than those "healthy" women who start showing in—*gasp!* their fifth month. Depending on what time of year you're pregnant, that can sit you out an entire bikini season (not even counting the months in hiding for that stubborn postpartum paunch). Other benefits of being a slimmer expectant? A thinner baby! Think about it. Baby will be one step closer to Hollywood's physical ideal right out of the womb. Besides, isn't it the responsibility of any mom to give her child an edge in life? The cutting-edge of fashion is no exception. But when is thin too thin? If you can make out baby's profile without the aid of an ultrasound, you might want to throw in an extra Slim-Fast on occasion.

Over-the-Hill Ovum

"I'm forty-two and after trying and trying, I'm finally pregnant. (And no, I didn't borrow someone's egg—I can barely bring myself to borrow a sweater.) I am worried about age and the risk to my baby. I'm also concerned about being an older parent."

Thanks to medical advances, your baby will likely be as healthy as one born to a twenty-five-year-old mother. Sure, your child may bear the stigma of having the only mom in a Hoveround at school functions (not to mention your MILF standing is long expired). That doesn't mean you can't be an effective parent. A young child will delight in swinging from your walker, and your teenager will love pilfering your overflowing medicine cabinet. The upside is you'll be too deaf, blind, and disoriented to know any better. Of course, there won't be a ton of parenting advice to be found in that large-print *Reader's Digest*—but who needs it when you have "Life in These United States"? Your children will also be young enough when you die to move into your spacious condo and throw some bitchin' parties. Coochie Coo? *Coo-coo-ca-choo!*

You've Got My Dinner in a Box

"My annoying neighbor told me that my microwave could be harmful to my unborn baby. But I just love that radioactive deliciousness—I have a Pavlovian response to the familiar beeping sounds. Still, should I get rid of ours for the duration of the pregnancy?"

You're right to be concerned. But don't throw the Hot Pockets out with your good sense. A microwave is a perfectly safe alternative to food preparation so long as you use precautions.

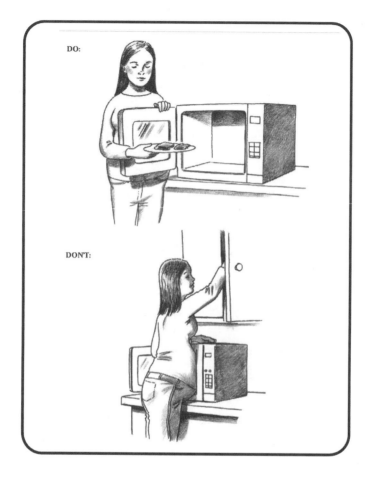

Other Unexpected Home Dangers

"We have a heated water bed, but, surprisingly, we're not in the porn industry. Will our sloshing sleep chamber put my baby at risk?"

I don't know which is more impressive. That you got enough traction on that thing to even get pregnant or that you've managed to go back in time twenty years. If you can simultaneously read and

OTHER HOUSEHOLD DO'S AND DON'TS

DO:

DON'T:

DO:

DON'T:

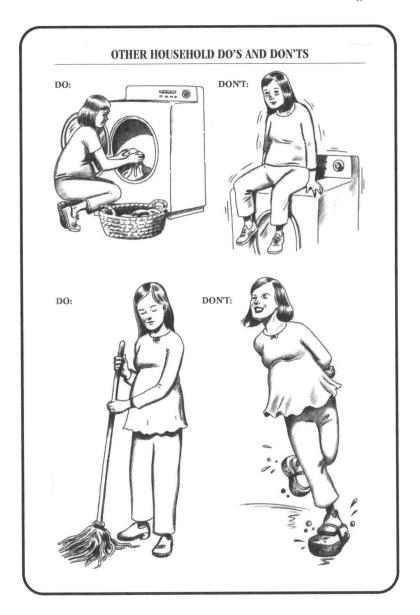

carry a boom box, I can tell you that, beyond your baby growing a mullet and wearing her onesie off a shoulder, the risk of water bed exposure is minimal. So the next time you're lying in bed, gazing at the reflection overhead, feel good about the person looking back at you. You're going to be a totally awesome parent. Just watch the comb in the back pocket.

Sliding Down the Corporate Ladder: How to Tell the Boss You've Got a New Boss

There's nothing supervisors like hearing more than that you're pregnant—especially male supervisors. While giving you a congratulatory hug, they can't help but note the potential sick days, the costly maternity leave, and the chilling reminder of what can happen when they bang the interns. You might feel a little nervous letting the head honcho know about your "woman's trouble." Fear not. Plenty of your fellow female co-workers have been there before.* Still, it might be best to wait a few months, to ensure all scheduled reviews and/or raises are in place. Below are some temporary concealment strategies until you're ready to make the big announcement.

In fact, navigating the workplace during your pregnancy might be the true test of your employer's family-friendly policies. For example, if you work at a successful dot-com, you'll likely be offered flextime, baby showers, and an office web-feed so your colleagues can watch the birth. On the other hand, if you work at a corporate law firm or financial institution, it's best to plant rumors that you're a drug addict to address any inconsistencies and avoid the stigma of being pregnant. Hints about a bulging

---

*See those passed over for promotion after promotion.

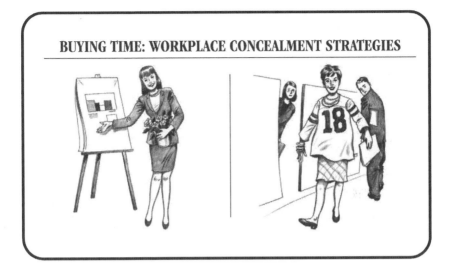

BUYING TIME: WORKPLACE CONCEALMENT STRATEGIES

tumor might also buy you some professional allowances. Remember, a tumor might go away; a baby won't.

How Pregnancy Can Be a Workplace Positive

Once it's clear to management that you don't have a tumor, and, instead, you're replicating, disappointment is bound to set in. This is when it's crucial to emphasize to the higher-ups how your condition will not only *not* interfere with your performance, but also how it can be an asset to the company as a whole. Here are some proposals to ease the boss's maternal misgivings.

- Insist on staying on the softball team. Advise that your delicate state will intimidate competitors from full-out play.
- Agree to neutralize any uncomfortable business dealings with "my water just broke"(later explained away with, "sorry, I just spilled my Sprite").

- Vow to hint aloud and often that the married rival CEO "may or may not" be the father.
- Propose shaving the company logo on the back of baby's head.
- Arrange to have the baby in the company lounge as a publicity stunt, proclaiming to all, "I wanted to give birth in the same place that gave me life."

How Women Handle the Big Announcement on the Job

- 10 percent told their boss immediately after finding out.
- 51 percent told trusted colleagues early and management after first trimester.
- 35 percent told no one until after the first trimester.
- 4 percent got outed by that bitch in accounting after vomiting in the bathroom.

CHAPTER 3

The First Trimester: The Long Road to a One-Piece Months One to Three

Welcome to the beginning of progressively getting fatter. The good news is, you have an entire trimester to still enjoy the land of the living before being immediately designated as "with child" or, alternatively, as an ineffective shoplifter. The bad news is, in those initial weeks, you'll have just enough paunch to look as though you're pregnant with, at most, a buffet. You may also experience nausea and occasional dizziness. If you aren't in the presence of Carrot Top, chances are your body is just reacting to hormone surges that are a normal part of early pregnancy.

PESTERING YOUR PRACTITIONER: WHAT HAPPENS AT THIS HOO-HA LOOK-SEE

Your initial prenatal physical exam will be the most uncomfortable you'll endure and even more so for the doctor assigned to your bottom half for the remainder of this vaginal journey. There are ways make things easier at both ends of the examining table. First, always practice good hygiene. If it looks like you've got Gene Shalit in a leg lock, you may want to clear a path, so to speak. Second, avoid any anecdotes that involve the phrases, "sue the pants off of..." or "my recent court settlement." Nothing turns a doctor off more, other than maybe the uninsured.

What's in There?

Even though you won't look pregnant those first few months, your clothes may be getting tighter around the middle. Your uterus has grown to the size of a small bunch of bananas (keeping with medicine's standardized fruit-size comparison scale. No "football-esque" or "miniature dog-like" references here!)

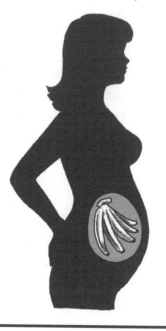

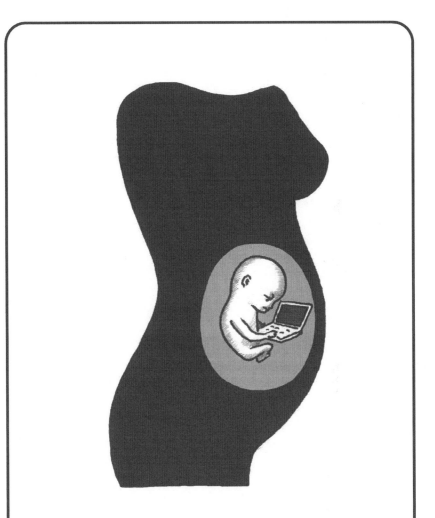

Over the first trimester, you baby will grow to a little over an inch long and, unlike your mother-in-law, will finally lose its tail. By the third month, baby is making spontaneous movements, like reading, checking email, and filling out change-of-address forms.

HOW PREGNANCY SCREWS WITH YOUR BODY AND MIND RIGHT NOW

PHYSICAL BREAKDOWN
- Bone-crushing fatigue
- *Thisclose* to peeing in pants all the time
- Nausea while reviewing current life standing
- Gas and swift social isolation

MENTAL DECLINE
- Joy
- Fear
- Confusion
- Contentment
- Anger
- Suicidal depression
- Back to joy

WHAT YOU MAY BE FREAKED OUT ABOUT
Rack Attack

"I've gone up two cup sizes, and I've only been pregnant for three weeks! Another month, and I'll be able to provide shaded parking."

Say hello to the breasts of a stripper and the bladder of a Shriner. Finally, a way to increase your bust without hating yourself enough to endure painful surgery! With your new, ample curves in place, you'll look hot for approximately one week, and half of that time will be spent racing back and forth to the toilet. Use the remainder wisely. Ask your male supervisor for that raise, get out of speeding tickets, and have your car serviced at generous discounts. For this brief window of time, the world is your double-D oyster.

Fearing Fallopian Faux Pas

"I have a friend who's desperately trying to get pregnant, but now I'm the one with the good news. I keep telling her it's as easy as penis in vagina—hello!?—but it doesn't seem to cushion the blow."

This is an awkward conversation, no matter how sensitive your approach. Here are some thoughtful ways to broach the topic, along with what *not* to say to your friend in-waiting.

Ways to preface the conversation:

Sensitive: "This might be hard for you to hear since you've been struggling…"

Insensitive: "This might be hard for you to understand since you're barren…"

Sensitive: "I hope you can find some happiness in what I'm about to tell you…"

Insensitive: "I hope you can finally find someone who can penetrate that fortress you call a cervix."

Sensitive: "I'm having a baby. I'll loan you my maternity clothes!"

Insensitive: "I'm having a baby. I'll loan you my husband since yours is obviously defective from the waist down."

Feline Not So Fine?

"My three cats rule the house. Despite this fact, I'm not crazy and, clearly, am sexually active. Will my unborn child contract toxoplasmosis from my pets? Should I give them away?"

Don't leave your kitties on the neighbor's doorstep with bows on their heads just yet. Your sharp-clawed companions have likely already given you toxoplasmosis years before, making you immune without you even knowing it. Sort of like that nasty rash your spouse said you caught from the toilet seat. So for now, your feline friends can stay put. As for giving your spouse away…now that's an idea you and your cats can get behind.

Electric Blanket Shocker

"My husband and I enjoy an electric blanket when it's cold out (making the wet spot that much more perilous). But what about now that I'm pregnant? Is an electric blanket bad?"

Unless you are a lizard and can't control your body's thermostat, there's really no need to bring a wire-lined blanket into bed with you. Just the pairing of the words "electric" and "blanket" alone are about as enticing a combo as "Tabasco" and "enema." Why not warm your slippers in a George Foreman grill or make your robe toasty over a space heater? When you get a chance, bring a lasagna over to the local fire station—oh, and maybe the blueprints of your house along with the number of people who generally sleep inside. No reason.

Unexpected Tips: Chill 101

One way to make sure you give your pregnancy the best chance is by finding ways to relax. But if you're like most mothers-to-be (or already a mom), you probably have very little time to unwind or are too uncool to score any of the hydroponic stuff. Here are some mini-escapes you can use throughout the day when anxiety strikes.

- Close your eyes. Imagine a beautiful scene—maybe an island getaway. Relax your muscles, starting from your feet to the legs, torso, neck, and face. Ignore all the honking and screaming and pleas that you're "going to kill someone." This is your moment.
- Inhale deeply and push your abdomen out as you do so. Let out a blissful sigh with each completion. Do ten times in a row—no matter what anyone at the meeting says.
- Find an isolated area, possibly at a nearby park. Give yourself fifteen minutes of alone time surrounded by nature. Disregard the wild dogs encircling you.

Haunted by the 90s...

"I can't help but worry that my wild party days of the past will cause me to lose the baby. In fact, Rick James once told me I needed to slow down. Is baby going to pay for my bad-girl ways?"

Fear not. If you're like most women, it's been years since you've huffed paint, not to mention that autoerotic suffocation was never your cup of tea. When it comes to being pregnant, here and now is all that matters. Your sins from the prenatal past aren't coming back to haunt you. So long as you're on a clean streak for the duration of the pregnancy, you have nothing to worry about except what color to paint the nursery (now without the euphoric hits to interrupt your progress!). Exception: if you slept with someone else's boyfriend or husband, and your current situation is that result. Then, boy oh boy, do you have it coming.

Pressure cooker Pregnancy

"My job is demanding—like Columbian drug lord/network executive demanding. Should I give notice now to protect the baby?"
If your job is stressful in that it's challenging, complex, and rewarding, then it's probably safe. If it's stressful as in dodging airborne objects or lying to Congress, then it might be better to opt out. Still, pregnancy can be a great buffer in those high-octane positions. Ways you can use your condition to your professional advantage? Cry when provoked. Cry when not provoked. Cry when your chips get stuck in the vending machine. When given bad news or poor performance evaluations, clutch your stomach and fall to the ground. Hello, extended paid maternity leave!

DAD'S HAVING A BABY TOO! MINUS ALL THE HARD STUFF
Your Partner in Pregnancy: That Bastard in the Barcalounger

Hey, you there, watching NASCAR. That's right, we haven't forgotten about the fathers along this extraordinary journey. Far from being left out, you're in luck: there isn't a chapter in this book that doesn't point out how this is all your fault! Remember, you poured the wine; you made the mix tape. Your involvement will be as natural as the responsibility required by your individual state.

It's Not About You Anymore, Pal

It might be hard to get a prospective dad excited about the months ahead when his progeny is only about as large as the very Cheetos that fuel him on a daily basis. Here are some visuals to help him imagine the possibilities to come.

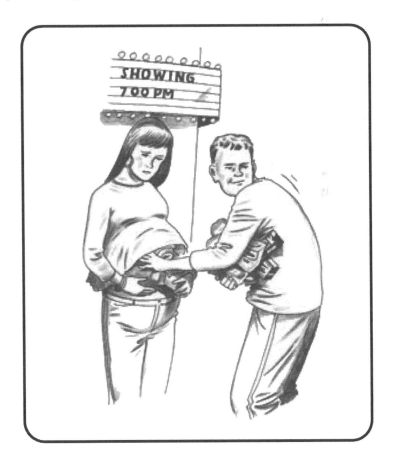

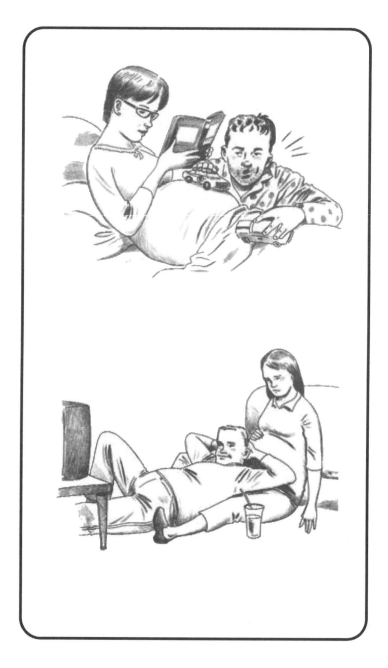

Remember Me? The One Who Got You Pregnant?

"My wife is so absorbed by the pregnancy that I feel left out. How can I make it all about me again?"

Wanting attention isn't selfish at all. It's perfectly normal to want to keep your spouse interested while having your own needs met. Here are some tips sure to spin her pregnant head around.

- Mention casually that Angelina Jolie was hot—until she polluted her uterus.
- Flirt with her childless friends. Comment aloud on their slim, non-childbearing hips.
- Leave computer window open to sites like "Hot Infertiles" or "Babes with No Stretch Marks."
- Masturbate shamelessly and often. When caught, calmly close the door and explain that she's "ruining it for you."
- Slowly drive by your old girlfriend's house—with her in the car.
- Take her to Hooters for lunch. Tell the buxom waitress you'll have "the usual."

Putting the "Ick" in Domestic: The Touchy-Feely Dad

While most women hope their partner will embrace the nine-month journey along with them, there is a small group of dads who take father prep to creepy, sensitive-guy extremes. When he's not serenading a cervix, he's posing for maternity pictures, gazing into his wife's stomach like a crystal ball. (The answer? Yes, you're a total douche.) A few pregnant women find this behavior endearing. Most, though, will tell you to just put your testicles in your handbag and make it official. Yes, you need to be involved, but if you use the words "mucus plug" as easily as you would the word "PlayStation," you've crossed the line, dude.

CHAPTER 4

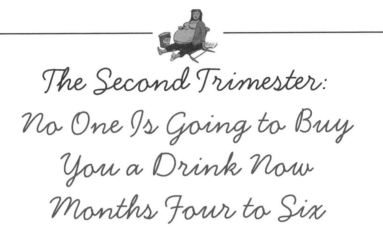

The Second Trimester: No One Is Going to Buy You a Drink Now Months Four to Six

These are the months when pregnancy will begin to seem real. You'll start to show and will finally conquer the coma-like fatigue and crushing depression that comes with early pregnancy.

PESTERING YOUR PRACTITIONER: WHAT HAPPENS AT THIS HOO-HA LOOK-SEE

- Much tsk-tsking over ballooning weight and sky-high blood pressure
- Dipping urine for sugar (not as delicious as it sounds)
- An ass-chewing for gaining too much weight

HOW PREGNANCY SCREWS WITH YOUR BODY AND MIND RIGHT NOW

PHYSICAL BREAKDOWN

- A level of exhaustion you never thought possible
- Less nausea (depending on who is present)
- Skin stretch rivaling that of comic-book superhero

MENTAL DECLINE
- Depression about showing and being classified on-sight as "the chunky friend"
- Volatility akin to unchecked bipolar disorder
- A feeling of being out of it—forgetting appointments, red lights, your pants

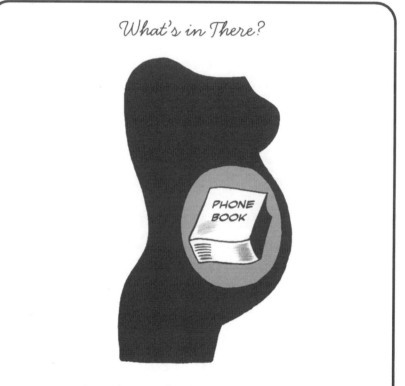

What's in There?

Your uterus is about the size of a phone book or a decapitated human head, whichever visual works for you. If you haven't told anyone about your pregnancy, rest assured the rumors are swirling and the "she so is" camp will finally be able to collect on their bets.

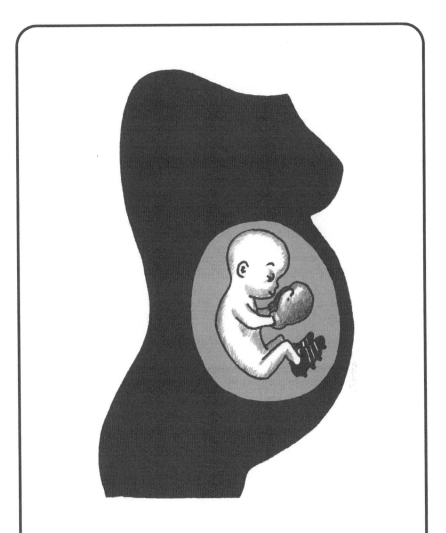

Your baby is getting longer (by the end of the second trimester, baby will be over two feet long and weigh up to five pounds—okay, no, but it feels like that) and is building strong bones, allowing her to randomly kick the crap out of you.

WHAT YOU MAY BE FREAKED OUT ABOUT
From Here to Maternity

"I can't fit into my jeans, but maternity wear costs more than the clothes I wore back when I looked good."

There's no reason to avoid clothes tailored for your bump. But if you can't see yourself in the expecting area of your local clothing outlet, there are temporary solutions to accommodate your growing girth. Ask that yo-yo dieter in your life for some hand-me-downs, or look for stores that have the word "woman" in the title. And remember, you don't have to be front and center at a Melissa Etheridge concert to don a pair of men's slacks. Elastic waistbands can also be a friend to an ever-expanding stomach. Just ask anyone exiting a Cracker Barrel.

It's a Boy...George?

Thanks to advances in modern technology, you can let the air out of one of nature's greatest surprises by finding out the gender through ultrasound. ("Hey everyone! It's a girl! Yeah, the same girl I told you about four months ago.") If you want to ensure a big *whatever* for your birth announcement, by all means, spill the beans. Nothing like the revelatory email that says, *Hey, those lungs have a ways to go, but baby has a discernible penis.* Another pitfall of putting your baby's genitals out there? You'll only get clothes at your shower. Horrible, horrible clothes: Grotesque tulle-ridden monsters and baby-blue short sets that would look gay on a gladiator. Do yourself a favor. Count the toes and fingers and concentrate on all returns you won't have to make.

He'd Better Get Used to Pink

"I feel terrible but as soon as I found out I was having a boy, I was let down. I hate football, not to mention that I've never even ridden in a truck."

It's normal to have a gender preference and feel a little taken aback when your daughter-to-be has a penis. In either case, you'll find both genders hold a wonder of unique experiences. One day, your baby boy will be all grown up and wrecking the car while your darling daughter will be webcasting her recently budded breasts. So enjoy the simplicity of either's early years. As for the boy blues, in a few months, you'll surely tire of tucking Timmy's wee-wee out of sight and dressing him like tea cozy. Meanwhile, Dad can help ease you into traditional boy activities while you reluctantly don a baseball glove and pray he turns out gay. If you're still feeling gypped by your XY standing, here are some effeminate-in-training techniques to make that boy a little more bearable.

- Affectionately refer to him as "girlfriend."
- When you wrap him in his blanket, barrage him with details of both blend and thread count.
- Tell him that onesie is really his color.
- Respond to his cries with "Don't go there."
- Occasionally warn that too much formula is going to go straight to his hips.

He'll be artfully arranging your antiques in no time.

I'll Tell You What I Should Have Told Him: Keep It to Yourself

"Now that it's clear I'm pregnant, every person I see insists on offering me tips. I may not remember where I parked these days, but I'm not stupid."

There's something about a pregnant belly that seems to attract every know-it-all in the country. Here are ways to make various advice-dispensers wish they had never laid eyes on your protruding profile.

- Reply loudly, "For the last time, the fetus is not for sale."
- Address public chidings about vigorous exercise or activity by calmly explaining you waited too long to "take care of the problem" so you're just giving Mother Nature a needed nudge.
- Sport horrific fake bruises on your face and arms and gush about how "the daddy was right about your willful ways."

This Test Is Open Book

"I'm over the age of thirty-five and was told I'd have to undergo a triple screen this month to test for genetic abnormalities. What can I expect?"

The triple screen is a blood test in which one sample can detect genetic abnormalities. What it can't test for are genetic aberrations like the propensity for back hair or online gambling. You're on your own there.

Ultra-Ultrasounds

"We recently saw a store at our mall that offered 4-D ultrasound images of your baby. Is this a good idea? We'd love to see if she's pageant material before the due date!"

Not to rain on your pre-peek parade, but it's a good rule of thumb to avoid medical practice within arm's reach of a Chick-fil-A. We realize the ability to buy a giant cookie, get your ears pierced, *and* see your infant in utero is a tempting combination, but try to resist. The sonographic training of the individuals operating these cervical glamour shots is probably not exactly in-line with AMA standards (and by AMA we mean American Medical Association, not American Mall Association). So skip "Fet-o-genic" or "Good Vibrations—Not to be Confused with the Sex Toy Store." Besides, you've got years to show off photos that no one but you cares about.

Triple Threat

"I'm pregnant with triplets. Against all advice, I've decided not to commit suicide and see the birth through. Will I have to have a cesarean?"

No, but it does mean your life is over. Don't believe it? Try carrying three bags of groceries. Mind you, these bags aren't screaming and gnawing at your shirt buttons, clamoring to be fed. It could be far worse, though. You could be one of those fertility freaks who gives birth to a family band only to end up having Diane Sawyer arrive at the crack of dawn to televise every stupid milestone. ("Look, little Jamie VI finally sprouted a tooth! Happy sixth birthday!") Parents of twins don't have it much easier. They have all of the multiple responsibilities and none of the glory. No one is stepping up to donate them a mega-house or commercial-sized washer. Twin parents face a life of doubled expenses along with economy-sized cereal boxes that, once empty (two days tops), can double as playhouse or spare bedroom. Don't laugh. The architects at General Mills will be your only savior.

Mood Swings: Welcome to the Personality Playground

During pregnancy, not only do you not feel like yourself phys-ically, but mentally, you're a stranger to boot. In a nutshell, you're an emotional rollercoaster; Sybil, but with larger breasts. But here's the good news. Pregnancy is a time in which violence is not only okay, it's natural and expected. Thanks to those swirling hormones, you've got a get-out-of-jail-free card—liter-ally. Your size alone is an intimidating factor. Shove a cop? That's a warning, Missy. You're just too adorable for a citation! Bitch-slap his ex? Smack away. What's she going to do? You've got a baby on board! Other *unexpected* outlaw recreations:

- Steal unabashedly. If caught, feign "mom brain."
- Cut in line at the bank, blaming your haste on contractions.
- Cry at the cosmetic counter about "feeling ugly" and receive a complimentary gift bag.
- Carjack with abandon. If caught, say you felt dizzy and were merely asking for a lift to the hospital.

PREGNANCY: A CORNUCOPIA OF SYMPTOMS

Getting bigger is only half the fun on this gestational joyride. Here are some common ailments along the nine-month sojourn that will make you positively nostalgic for a hangover.

Morning Sickness: Hugging a Surface That Had an Ass on It

For most, morning sickness is just a convenient way to shed those pounds that you should have lost before the pregnancy. With the sense of smell equal to that of a purebred dog, you can now process every wretch-inducing aroma around you. Who knew a whiff of water could be so objectionable? Still, if you're puking like a ballet dancer well into the second trimester, consider it a dress rehearsal for your post-birth weight-loss plan.

Rip Van Winkle-Like Fatigue

If you've never been unemployed, this is what it feels like. The couch will be your newfound lover, the only one who truly understands you. The little time you'll spend apart from your sectional soul mate will likely be motivated by the ocean of urine that now makes up your entire lower quadrant. In most cases, fatigue will lift after the second trimester, not too far before hourly waking and feedings will make you envy a sleep-deprived prisoner in Guantanamo.

Round-Ligament Pain: Your Inner Taser

Feel like you've been gutted by a serrated knife in your lower abdomen? That's round-ligament pain, a lightning-like abdominal jolt that will teach you never to do something as frivolous as sneeze or stand again. Round-ligament pain often traces the same area where your bikini would follow—not that you'll be wearing one ever again.

A Runny Nose

Now that you're pregnant you no longer get your period. Instead, your nose has one! With blood vessels pumping more and more blood, you too can look like you're engaged to a 'roid-raging professional athlete.

Yeast Infections

Feeling as itchy as a ballplayer? It's not uncommon to suffer a yeast infection during pregnancy, due to increased estrogen levels. The cure: try an over-the-counter treatment, wear breathable underwear, and don't host any bake sales.

Gas/Heartburn

And you just thought you weren't hot. With you're new intestinal fortitude, you're like a guy, but without the penis or higher income. If your hormones haven't shredded the last remains of your relationship, sleeping in that Dutch oven you call a bed will finish off the rest.

PREGNANCY AS A FASHION/PERSONAL STATEMENT

Long gone are the days of the arrow "baby" T-shirt. Now, you can dress as slutty as you did in college. Today, a pregnant belly is hardly a fashion impediment. In fact, the pregnancy itself can be *tres chic*, not to mention a publicity one-two punch for the eating disorder/drug habit combo. One week, you're wasted; next week, *empire*-waisted! But pregnancy isn't just about Pucci dresses, ballet flats, and lies. It's about getting lots of attention for opening your legs at the right time. If famous, or just unhappy in general, consider maximizing your pregnancy press with a self-styled exposure video ("Mamas Gone Mad") or start a children's foundation where you own offspring will inevitably seek asylum.

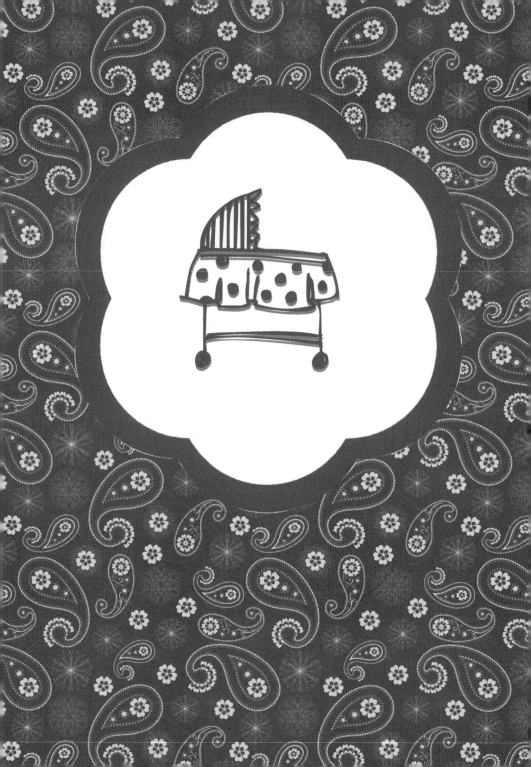

CHAPTER 5

The Third Trimester: "Wow. You're, Like, Huge." Months Seven to Nine

You're nearing the finish line and are likely getting anxious about evicting that little uterine tenant. Like a lot of bad boarders, he or she is probably making a ruckus at all hours. In this case, pounding you with little feet and stabbing you with what feels like an anorexic's elbows. But it's not just your insides that are being turned upside down. With a baby imminent, your day-to-day surroundings are subject to overhaul. At home, safety will be most prominent in your decorating scheme. For example, your floating glass coffee table will now be anchored with Nerf-like bumpers, and opening cabinets will require an engineering degree. But how do you know that you've met all hazard-proof requirements? If you pee yourself while trying to safe-crack your toilet, you should be covered.

PESTERING YOUR PRACTITIONER: WHAT HAPPENS AT THIS HOO-HA LOOK-SEE
- Mouth-dropping weigh-in
- The usual battery of tests and annoyance at your "I'm in labor!" paranoia

HOW PREGNANCY SCREWS WITH YOUR BODY AND MIND RIGHT NOW

PHYSICAL BREAKDOWN

- Baby kicking like David Beckham
- Breasts that could suffocate a small child
- Gross protruding navel

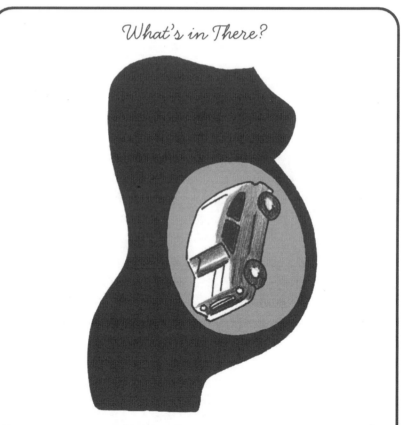

What's in There?

Your uterus can now house a Fiat. Interesting pregnancy trivia: The measurement from the top of your pubic bone to the top of your uterus correlates to the number of weeks you're up to (36 centimeters=36 weeks). Your final week's measurement also corresponds into the number of years until you get a peaceful night's sleep again.

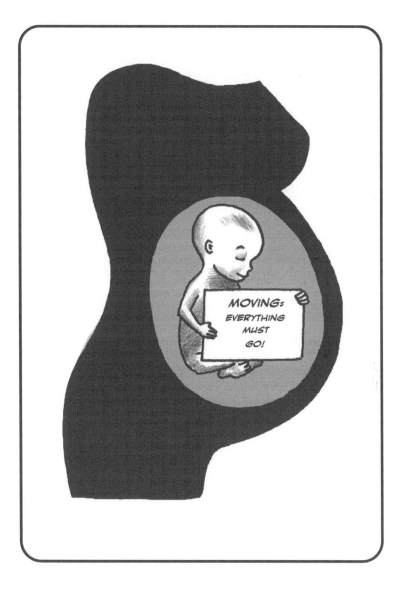

MENTAL DECLINE

- Excitement about meeting your little passenger, followed by utter dismay about how she plans on getting here

WHAT YOU MAY BE FREAKED OUT ABOUT
Einstein in Utero

"I read that listening to classical music will make a baby musically gifted. Can I create a musically inclined baby even if I didn't sleep with John Tesh?"

The idea that music makes baby into a Mozart is no more true than the idea that listening to your latest argument with your husband will make her a marriage therapist. In fact, it's important to know that fetuses often have a different sleeping pattern than you, so unless you'd love to hear *Beowulf* at 3 a.m., keep the ambush reading sessions to a minimum. Some studies show that the sound of the mother or father's voice is particularly soothing to the infant, since the little darling hears both on a regular basis before birth. If you don't feel too odd talking to your bloated abdomen, here are some great in-utero conversation starters:

- "Hot enough for ya?"
- "Ready to save Mommy's marriage?"
- "My love for you—and for the monthly checks you've ensured—is very real."
- "I didn't get to be a model or be a child actor. Rest assured, I won't let that happen to you."

Unexpected Sex: Baby, I'm Knocking at the Door but Please Don't Answer

Sex during pregnancy can be a confusing time for any couple. You may still have the same desires of a woman half your size, while your husband should be nominated for an Academy Award for his ability to obtain an erection in your presence. Also, bouts of fatigue and nausea and breasts with the pain index of gigantic testicles aren't exactly romantic mood enhancers. Here are some common pregnancy sex concerns and why you should put those worries in bed to bed.

AFRAID OF INJURING BABY AND/OR BABY UNDERSTANDING

No chance. Your fetus is highly protected by an amniotic sac and completely oblivious to the coital coupling. It's just you, your husband, and your God watching—and judging.

AFRAID THAT ORGASM WILL START LABOR

Another one to put on the not-to-worry list. It's been *years* since he's given you an orgasm.

PARENTAL YUCK FACTOR

You both may be adjusting to your changing roles. Try to concentrate on the fact that sex is now purely recreational and free of planning or procreating detail. But be patient. After all, he is doing it with a mom.

Not-So-Hot Mama

"My wife is very pretty while pregnant, but, still, she's pregnant. Eww. As for sex, I can only keep suggesting 'from behind' for so long."

Some men find the pregnant body erotic. Others consider it a flesh-and-blood reminder that vaginas aren't just fun pockets: babies come out of them. In either case, it's crucial that your wife feels desired during her delicate state. If it helps, think of her stomach as an extra boob. Or maybe, have sex in the shower with the curtain as a handy divider. See, those Hasidic Jews are onto something!

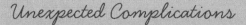

Unexpected Complications

Bed Rest

At some point along the pre-term trail, you may find yourself assigned to bed rest, which is basically a license to get fat. While your body remains immobile, your ability to burn calories will be restricted to desperately clicking your weak-signaled remote before—ahhhhh!—having to watch *Tyra*! Once you've avoided a close encounter of the "girlfriend!" kind, you've still got another twenty-three-and-a-half hours left to watch your ass grow. Here's how you can fill the time while you and baby are stranded on mattress island.

- Send your partner to buy a *TV Guide* and, armed with high-lighter, plot out your week's television viewing. If you're feeling undermined by your terrycloth attire, feel free to note "appointments" in your BlackBerry or day planner. For example: 9 a.m.: Gab with Regis, endure Kelly; 12 p.m.: Find the real Salem killer; 3 p.m.: Solve an *Unsolved Mystery* from 1987; 4 p.m.: Run around barefoot with Inga; 5 p.m. Detox with CNN and play anchor matchmaker—Lou Dobbs? Fredricka Whitfield!

- If in viewing distance of neighbors, make up wild, *Rear Window*-like tale for spouse upon return home from work. Once you've convinced him the neighbor's wife is now fortifying their prize-winning azaleas, casually dismiss the allegations, saying you "probably dreamed it."
- Make a culinary trip around the world via take-out. Divide your bed into various flavorful countries. Next stop? Italy/pillow shams!
- Commandeer husband's laptop and scan his bookmarks. Replace each yank-time favorite with a link to remind him of you: Breast Fest 2008 becomes Recipes.com; Mistress Mindy's Dungeon becomes Ann Taylor Loft.

A Threesome—Not the cool Kind

"My desire is still there, but my stomach literally gets in our way. My husband doesn't even know where to aim anymore."

Far from pushing you apart, pregnancy can be a great time to reinvigorate your love life. Use your creativity! There are some positions men tend to prefer but are afraid to express to their partner. Favorites include in front of the computer while you're out running errands and in the shower when you finally give the man five minutes of peace.

WE DON'T NEED NO EDUCATION
Instruction/Birthing Classes: Giving New Meaning to the Term "Slasher Film"

Do you like watching violent porn? How about with lots of strangers in the room? Expect a similar level of comfort when entering the realm of the birthing class. From the onset, you're told it's a great way to meet other couples in the same birthing boat. In reality, you don't want friends who aren't smart enough to skip it.

If you're foolish enough to stick it out, you get what you deserve: namely, the child-birthing video. From the team that brought you *Faces of Death* comes the tale of your tail, wrecked beyond all imagination. You'll wax sentimental for those gratuitous beheadings and eviscerations once you see a head tearing its way though that 70s-coifed mons pubis. Trust us, Rob Zombie has nothing on the folks at Emerging Life Films.

The information you need is pretty simple, really. Whether you're of the Alexander, Bradley, or the Bite-a-Rope-and-Curse school, the rundown will be the same: a human being is going to (a) emerge from your vagina; or (b) be airlifted from your stomach by forceps. There's going to be torn flesh; there's going to be pain. People are going to say and do stupid things throughout the entire process. Everyone will annoy you. You will look like a sea lion in all pictures. *Tada*, you're a mom.

Congratulations: you just saved yourself a few hundred dollars and six weeks of your life.

child care Education: Stupidity with a Syllabus

Many hospitals offer baby-care classes to help expectant moms and dads prepare for their new roles once their little one is here. You may want to consider baby-care education, especially if you found eighth-grade hygiene class enlightening. Instructional gems include not disposing of your infant in the trash and fastening the diaper on the end that doesn't scream.

Of course, recent parolees and crackheads will be all ears, furiously scrawling notes on the back of paper sacks or the canvas of their open palm. You, on the other hand, may feel the lessons are somewhat intuitive, as demonstrated by the below sample syllabus. Student comments in italics:

Month One: Officially Pregnant
Tell everyone at school I'm getting fat.
Month Two: Making Financial Arrangements
Extort baby's daddy.
Month Three: Diet Concerns
Switch from MacDonald's to Taco Bell Fresco menu.
Month Four: Invoking Good Habits
Stop smoking—weed.
Month Five: Enforce Discipline
Stop drinking—in the morning.
Month Six: Limiting Stressful Physical Activities
Stop stealing cars and switch to insurance scams.
Month Seven: Practical Matters
Accept the pregnancy.

Month Eight: Nursery Prep
Pick a drawer for baby's bed.
Month Nine: Labor And Deliver
Attend prom.

Another hundred dollars saved.

CHAPTER 6

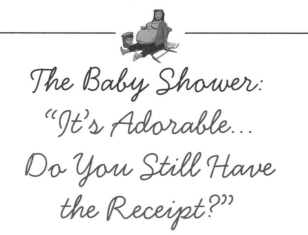

The Baby Shower: "It's Adorable... Do You Still Have the Receipt?"

If you've ever used the term "Aunt Flo" for your period or if you own a festive holiday sweater, chances are the baby shower will be one big orgasm for you and your kind. For the rest, it will be just another uncomfortable rite of pregnancy along with hemorrhoids and chapped nipples. If you aren't exactly ready to jump into the cult of crustless sandwiches, here are some pointers to help you fake it while amongst the blue and pink believers.

HOW PREGNANCY SCREWS WITH YOUR BODY AND MIND RIGHT NOW

PHYSICAL BREAKDOWN

- Nausea
- Dread

MENTAL DECLINE

- Nervousness that people will show up and make you go through with this

- Increased anxiety as nothing is purchased from your on-line registry

WHAT YOU MAY BE FREAKED OUT ABOUT
Invitations

As mentioned, pink and blue are ideal, but bonus points for storks, ducks, or other animals that make up the curious marriage of babies and nit-covered wildlife. Rhyming invitations are especially appreciated. Examples can include: *There's a new baby on the way; Come and join our special day* while avoiding any verses that point out the delicate or obvious: *Have your cake and get your fill; Marcia forgot to take her pill.*

Picking a Theme

Today's modern shower sect isn't happy with just cake, punch, and presents. Your impending baby party must have a theme in order to truly legitimize your pregnancy. Otherwise, you're just another uterus in use. Popular objectives include limiting your future daughter to frilly, traditional roles or turning your son-in-waiting into a gay sailor. Conversely, themes like *Let's Get This Over With (That's What She Said)* and *Abortion Wasn't an Option* might cast a pall on your fetal festivities.

Games

Forced merriment wouldn't be complete without the introduction of games too infantile for even the gestational guest of honor. If you've ever willingly teetered an egg and spoon in your mouth or raced in a sack without the influence of alcohol, you'll be in hokey heaven. If you just can't stand the thought of "Bobbing for Binkies," though, here are some unique competitions that will make your shower one they'll never forget. (Not to mention you may never be asked to attend or host another in your life.) Nontraditional alternatives include:

- *Guess the Secret Infertile*
- *Who Weighs More than the Mom?*
- *Bastard? Not a Bastard?*
- *Does He Still Hit That?*
- *What Can She Hold Under Her Breasts?*
- *Placenta Recipe Swap*

More Ways to Get Your Game On

Traditional favorites: Old-wives'-tale games for guessing the sex

If you didn't find out the sex of the baby, you're going to be punished appropriately: enter old-fashioned gender guessing games.

These are usually initiated by the oldest guest at the party (the one who will buy you everything from Carter's) and will cause you to question if this is a shower or a Wicca membership drive. The rites of passage for gender play vary from the benign (hanging crystals over the belly) to the extreme (levitation and ritualistic killings. Hey, what did you think the duckies and bunnies were for?) Others may want to guess the sex based on your shape and the way you carry. If you thought you were self-conscious before, see how you feel once you've been group-diagnosed with the unmistakable wide girth that points to boy or the low, dumpy belly indicative of a girl. Above all, try to remember it's all in good fun—if you manage to draw the line in time at breast density assessment.

Gifts: The Art of Not Acting Disappointed

What you can expect to get at a baby shower? Weeks before, you will have probably entered the exciting realm of the baby registry. This is a ritual that allows you to go to your favorite store and hand-pick and fondle all the gifts you hope to receive but won't. More specifically, it is the place where hope dies. That's because everyone has her own idea of what's best for baby and mom and, in most cases, it's got Winnie-the-Pooh written all over it. Returns, you might ask? Not if it's bought at Babies-R-From-Heaven boutique in Wichita, Kansas. That swing you ordered? Surprise! It's a clown lamp! The designer "Pack 'n Play" you've been lusting after? Meet "Stow 'n Sleep," its cheap and evil cousin—likely from your cheap and evil cousin. But as much as you might be disappointed in the quality of loot, feigning appreciation is must. After all, one-armed sweaters don't knit themselves. Below are some go-to gratitude one-liners to help you describe the indescribable:

- "I can't believe you found a matching necklace, bracelet, ring, toe ring, earring, charm, and anklet set all in her birthstone. Who's the classiest baby now?"
- "A baby headband—in rhinestones! Add a matching teething grill, and I'll be the envy of all the moms in Compton!"
- "Goodness! A membership in the NRA! I've always thought of Charlton Heston as a grandfatherly figure."

- "A lotion warmer. Thank you! What great multipurpose gift! For K-Y, maple syrup…"
- "*Aww*. A 'Jesus Loves Me' bear. Now all the kids in Temple will want one!"

BABY GEAR: WHAT YOU'LL REGISTER FOR BUT HAVE TO BUY YOURSELF…

After you emerge from that pile of awful baby clothes and nothing else, you'll have a list a mile long of things to buy that you can actually use. So what's all this stuff for anyway?

Strollers: Baby's First Status Symbol

Your baby may be too young to drive, but they're never too young to be judged. Enter the uber-stroller. Equipped with exotic names and impressive turn radii, they sport most every modern convenience except a place to store a diaper bag or set a drink.

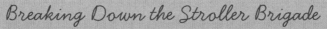

Breaking Down the Stroller Brigade

The mom behind the wheels

EXPENSIVE CELEBRITY STROLLER

This mom loves Victoria Beckham and/or Sarah Jessica Parker and would wear her skin if she could. Her secret dream is to have one of her "whimsical" (read: professionally planned six months in advance) kids' parties featured in a lifestyle magazine or become a children's clothing designer. She has a piece of baby bling for every child she pushed out of her five-carat vagina. Her hobbies include antiquing, evaluating preschools, and vomiting.

THE JOG STROLLER

Always in a ponytail and jog bra—even if not jogging. Her grip is almost as tight as her smile as she silently critiques every mom who dares to amble at a normal pace. She speaks of carbs as someone else might speak of Al Qaeda. (Note: Her seemingly peacefully sleeping child has actually been jostled unconscious.) Her hobbies include running. Only running.

THE NON-CONVERTIBLE PRAM

She really, *really* wanted to get pregnant and just spent a grand on a stroller with three months' use, max. She'll spend triple that on couples' therapy to mend the relationship with the invisible jerk lagging ten feet behind her now that "the love of her life" is finally here. Her hobbies include baby scrapbooking, mommy blogging, and entering her child in online photo contests.

FOLD AWAY STROLLER

She's on her fourth kid and would be just as happy tying baby to a rolling suitcase and herself to a rolling car. She has horse-tail-length hair and bangs that never grow. She owns a Crock-Pot and uses it. She'll make you go to theme and chain restaurants that feature animatronic animals. Her hobbies include converting strangers and selling Amway.

(Reason goes that if you're pushing a $900 stroller, you can likely employ someone to hold both.) Some manufacturers go as far as to call their carting contraptions "Infant Systems" and claim to "last a lifetime." As if one day, your college-bound Janie will use those shock-absorbing wheels to navigate uneven campus terrain. In fact, the real endorsement for such an exorbitant purchase is rarely, if ever, highlighted; namely, to keep lesser mothers from invading your social circle. With on-sight socioeconomic classification, you won't waste time befriending someone who doesn't have a pool or a vacation home that might benefit you and your family. Think that Baby-Bargain cart hauler is going to be a good reference for an exclusive preschool? Ignore such indicators and suffer the consequences of hand-me-down requests and play dates at McDonald's.

And There's More...

Take a look at some of the obvious and not-so-obvious applications for the baby utilities that you'll eBay those knitted booties to afford.

BABY MONITOR:
For hearing baby from other rooms and accidentally broadcasting your latest spousal fight to everyone downstairs.

BREAST-FEEDING PILLOW:
For around-the-waist breast-feeding and around-the-ass cushioning while the "garage" is in disrepair.

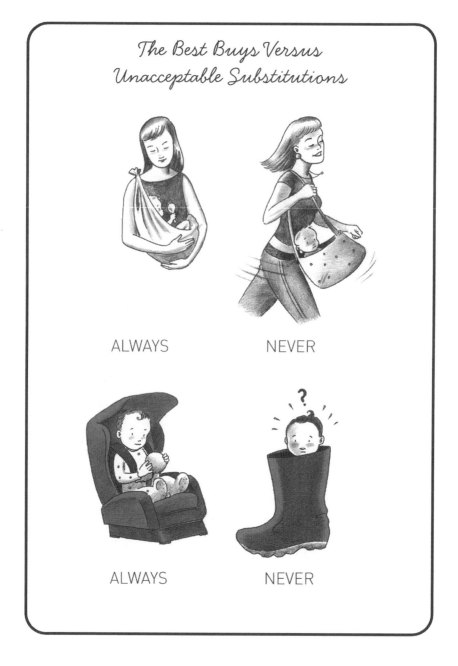

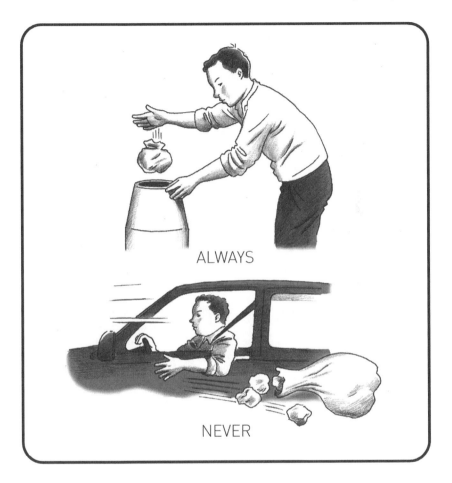

ALWAYS

NEVER

WRAP-EM TIGHT BLANKET:

For comforting baby or restraining mom during violent post-partum episode.

RUB-A-DUB TUB:

For taking up the entire space of your own bathtub until you realize the sink is just as good.

EXERCISE MAT:

To improve motor skills and hand-eye coordination while enticing housecats to a swat duel with baby.

EDUCATIONAL DVDS:

For introducing baby to songs, shapes, and other visual interests while Mommy and Daddy make a comical attempt at sex.

CAR SEAT:

For ensuring baby's safety in transit and through its unbelievably difficult installation, reminding you that you'd never cut it as a single mom.

The Shower's Torturous Hybrid: The Office Shower

There's nothing like hosting an event at your workplace that forces your colleagues to acknowledge your vagina. The office shower brings a new level of discomfort to workplace politics: think pap smear and annual review combined. Unlike the rabid attendees at a personal shower, the office shower will be as mercifully short as your post-birth career. Decorations will consist of whatever was available at the local Rite-Aid—so don't be surprised if future baby gets welcomed with "Luck o' The Irish" or "A Very Hoppy Easter" well into the fall. This party will result in your worst gifts yet. If the attendees even know your last name, they certainly haven't glanced at the registry; most just were unwittingly lured into the conference room by the smell of food. Don't be surprised if baby gets that paper clip mobile or handy eraser teether you've been dreaming about. And it goes downhill from there. Specifically, the only thing more humiliating than stepping into the office elevator carrying a diaper cake will be toting that medieval-looking device known as a breast pump in the months ahead. *Say, what is that?* asks Ron from accounting. Doors close.

Leave Your Manhood at the Door: The couples' Shower

Somewhere along the line, some idiot man with enough sperm to get a woman pregnant, but not enough to save himself, said, *Gee, I want to be part of the fun.* This moron has been on every man's hit list since. He's the same guy that forced "we're pregnant" into male mouths and probably invented the carryall "Diaper Dude." For women, he is a godsend, allowing the baby shower to become not much more than a benign barbeque attended by the most whipped men to ever procreate. Still, as much as they would like to pretend otherwise, this is a shower and somewhere along the line, emasculating games must occur. Most of the male attendees will turn to alcohol to numb the pain of participation. On the other hand, if your guy relishes "pass the pacifier" or is first in line to belly cast, you may want to save some of that papier mâché to spackle your vagina shut permanently after the baby is born.

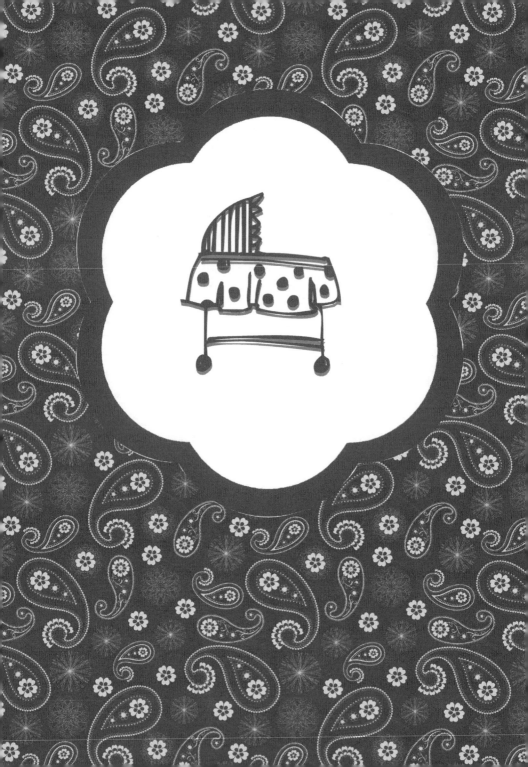

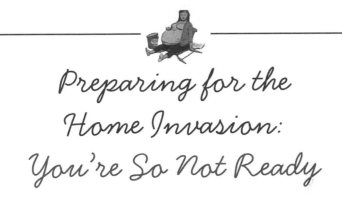

CHAPTER 7

Preparing for the Home Invasion: You're So Not Ready

THE UNHERALDED ART OF BABY PROOFING

Time to face reality. Those carefree days of toasting bagels mid-bath are over. Even though your little one won't be crawling for some months, it's wise to make preparations now before junior decides to navigate the electrical closet or gnaw on some toys made in China.

Unexpected ideas:

- Applying corner bumpers to protect against falls and to leave a permanent resin on your precious antiques, gently reminding you of infanthood should you ever dare to want another child.

- Enjoying your thin and childless friends whom you will not be able to tolerate once the baby is born.

- Installing doorway gates to corral baby and cause you to break your neck while trying to step over it with a load of laundry. (Loud slamming or clicking sounds of latch also doubles as a mommy motion detector should you ever try to slip out of the room while baby sleeps.)

- Adding cabinet locks to make you think twice about whether or not you really want that snack, and for leaving sitters and houseguests to starve when you leave and inevitably forget to tell them how to operate. ("It's easy. Just put the little magnetic handle up against the cabinet door until you hear a 'click.' It won't unlock, but that means you've found the inner hardware. Use the magnet to trace tiny little circles on the outer surface directly in line with where the inner cabinet latch should be. Then use this stethoscope to try to hear the latch detach. If it does, immediately pull the cabinet handle, and if it's meant to be that you should obtain entry, it will happen!"

- Installing pool netting as safety layer as well as backdrop for bad-ass Spider-man impressions.

- Using toilet locks to keep baby from falling in and for practicing your own postpartum bladder control.

- Beeping door alarms to alert for baby headed outdoors or spouse sneaking out for a smoke.

THE PARANOID PREGNANCY: MERCURY, LEAD, AND ARTIFICIAL SWEETENERS, OH MY!

Sure, pregnancy takes all the fun out of eating disorders, but for the obsessive-compulsive, it's a carnival of procreative precautions. Disinfectant wipes? Check. Liquid hand sanitizer? Check. Blood sample for unsafe ammonia levels? Check. Tired of feeling weird about saving your urine in jars? Who isn't? Don't worry— whoops—*do* worry. It's okay. You're pregnant!

For the paranoid mom, pregnancy is one big Petri dish of disastrous possibilities. One cup of coffee and you've got a lazy eye, or an extra set of genitals to powder and diaper. For you, a glass of wine might as well be strychnine, bug repellant, napalm. That breath-sucking cat? To the pound! Besides, who are these soft-cheese eating mothers and where is CPS when you need them?

when Your Paranoia and Your Doctor collide

The paranoid preggy either: (a) hates doctors and trusts no one affiliated with a medical facility; or (b) loves doctors and enjoys regaling them with every vaginal discharge anecdote they can muster. The former group will rely either on family for medical guidance, or on a woman dressed like Stevie Nicks who holds a continuing-education degree.

If you're of the latter group, though, the doctor visit is the highlight of your month and will generally go as follows: ob-gyn will approach exam-room door. On the other side, you'll hear them flipping the pages of your chart, then letting out a giant sigh. The door will swing open with all the momentum it takes for your doctor to face another hour of "what's that discharge/belly flinch/pelvic pain." Your legs will go into stirrups and your gown will conceal their dead eyes as they spelunk into your average vagina as perfunctorily as the act that got you there in the first place. "Okay, everything looks fine," they will say, and they mean it, but you won't be dismissed that easily. Twelve years of specialized schooling is one thing, but can it really compare with the immediacy and accuracy of information on the Web? The questions will start to roll and, on cue, the nurse enters.

"You're needed in Room 2," she says to the doctor. Before you can wield your printouts, the white coat is a blur. The door shuts. High-fives are exchanged.

Feeling paranoid now?

Paranoid Baby Prep

BASSINET OR WICKER COFFIN? YOU BE THE JUDGE...

Getting ready for baby can present numerous challenges. Particularly if, for you, morbidity and maternity go hand-in-hand. For a paranoid preggy, getting ready for baby is like a nine-month episode of *Looney Tunes* featuring Wile E. Coyote and Road Runner, and every nursery product has ACME written all over it. Changing tables are potential cliff falls; that baby chandelier, a crystal-adorned anvil. So how do you know when you're stepping into Howard Hughes territory when it comes to parenting paranoia? Tell-tale clues:

Normal: Lysol wipes
Not normal: Boric acid wipes

Normal: Rail guards to protect baby
Not normal: *Real* guards to protect baby

Normal: Sleep monitor
Not normal: Cardiac monitor

THE NAME GAME: FRUIT OR ACTION VERB?

Joe and Jane, where have you gone? Certainly not to the pages of *US Weekly*, the new name resource when it comes to inflicting shame for a lifetime. Celebrities have long gone out of their way to protect animals from cruelty but draw a firm line in the case of naming their offspring. Who needs the plight of the chinchilla when you've got "Pilot" or "Racer?"

Gwyneth inspired thousands of wannabes to turn to their fruit bowls when she chose the simple but controversial "Apple." But everyday followers of such unique monikers forget that celebrity children are insulated by a last name—a *famous* last name. "Apple Martin? Right this way!" "Apple Horowitz?" Not so much. So if you aren't screwing someone with a SAG card, think practicality. Remember, "Peaches" may be adorable on a cherubic six-month-old, but ask Peaches about it when she's trying to make partner.

We can also credit celebrity culture for helping us to look to various states and basic nouns as name inspiration. Don't worry. "Door" will learn to thank you for those character-building beatings by "Hemp" and "Gauge" who are just turning their own rage out on wussier-named children. "Flower," can you say "homeschool?" Sadly, there are throngs of sheep just waiting to follow suit.

Hey. "Sheep"…

Name as a Destiny

When parents bestow a chosen moniker upon their child, they also bestow potential life experiences. For example, a Jake or William might likely be tapped for the big promotion, while a

Chester might get tapped by the bigger guy in the adjoining cell. At the same time, names with unique spellings or double meanings might require you to make your child's future résumé flame retardant. "X-tee" (Christie) has an excellent chance of that second-round interview so long as the job requires negative blood tests and an explicit jpeg. So when you're sitting around with your spouse mulling potential names, think about what future Internet results you want for your kid's name: *Forbes's* List of Philanthropic Billionaires, or porn pop-ups?

Handy At-a-Glance Name Guide

NAMES TO FACILITATE A CAREER IN PORN
Amber
Ebony
Derrick
Nikki
Rick

NAMES TO ENSURE HOMEBODY STATUS
Alice
Edwin
Roger
Carol
Kathy*

*Highest chance of cat ownership

NAMES TO ENSURE HILLBILLY STATUS
For girls, anything paired with Lynn, Ann, or Sue
For boys, Junior. Period.

NAMES TO FACILITATE A LIFE OF CRIME
Anything paired with "Wayne" or "Ray" = serial killer

"But I Like Gertrude:" Coming to a Compromise

Choosing a name both you and your partner like can be especially difficult. When it comes to girls, moms often choose names they can identify with, whereas dads tend to lean toward names of ex-girlfriends whom they cannot forget. For boys, a woman may love a unique name that makes him stand out from the crowd, while the man sees him standing out from the crowd and being pantsed. Family names can also be a sticking point. You may want to pass along Grandmother Elizabeth's fine name, but will you be able to shake the image of her snacking out of the dog's bowl?

If you can't decide who gets to make the final call, defer to the person who's chosen the closest human names for pets in your family. (And they laughed when you named your cat Catherine Zeta-Jones!)

Sharing the Name with Others before the Birth: Keep Your Damn Mouth Shut

"What are you going to name the baby?"

"Theodore."

"There was a Theodore in our neighborhood. He used to touch himself while waiting for the bus."

Told you. Shut it.

Outwitting the Name Naysayers

Surprisingly, there will be several difficult people to navigate during this seemingly benign rite of pregnancy. Here are a list of possible saboteurs who feel entitled to title your baby.

THE NOT-EVEN-PREGNANT NAME HOARDER

You share your hopes for little Eva only to be confronted with, "That's my name!" Unbeknownst to you, this person, still menstruating on a regular basis, copyrighted the moniker and expects you to abide by the laws of "called it" despite her babyless status. Even though she may or may not ever give birth, you're nothing less than a total bitch if you tread anywhere near the rightful appellation of her child, currently consisting of stardust. Here's a name for you: *crazy*.

THE OLD PERSON TRYING TO FIND MEANING IN HIS DISAPPOINTING LIFE

And guess where they plan to find it? Right on your child's birth certificate. This is usually a man in the family who treated you like garbage up to the point he saw your prospective child as a gateway to his immortality. Remind Gramps or Uncle Albert he could have had his name on any building or park had he done something worth a damn. Worst case, name the family dog after him and call it even.

The Breast

Food or Fondling

This is the question faced by anyone considering breast-feeding. For many, the transition of turning an object of sexuality into something as utilitarian as a beverage fountain can be somewhat disorienting. Possibly no different than if your pubic region suddenly doubled as a nacho bar or reservoir for salad fixings. But can you still find erotic pleasure in something that now has a practical purpose? One possible solution can be to designate a feeding boob and a "bad" boob, the one to which your husband can lay filthy claim. Like a set of evil and good twins, they can work in oppositional concert, bringing balance to your baby, your husband, and the universe as a whole.

WHY SOME PREFER THE BOOB

- It's great if you want to bond as closely with your baby as possible or are downright poor.
- Because it requires more advanced work of the palate, baby is finally doing his share.
- It's an easy way to get men's attention while still being out of shape.

WHY SOME PREFER THE BOTTLE

- Doesn't allow infant to get too "reliant" or "clingy" in case things don't work out between you.
- No risk of leaky gaskets during sex.
- Instantly cooler than moms who breast-feed.

SMOKING AND BREAST-FEEDING: YOU'VE COME A LONG WAY, BABY

- Because nicotine does pass through the breast milk (and fontanel indention does make for a tempting ashtray) quitting smoking is ideal. Not to mention your good example might put off baby's habit for at least another twelve years.

THE CRITIC

(Also refer to above section, "Keep Your Damn Mouth Shut.") You like Helen. "But people will call her 'Hel' for short," says this annoying little voice of dissent. Harry? "Uh...*Hairy* like an ape. Please!" This person is likely a reformed playground masochist, the one who taunted even the most commonly dubbed child to distract from, oh, say, the fact her mother showed up drunk at PTA meetings. No matter the suggestion, she will assure you that your child is doomed to ridicule if you dare to go the way of Jane or John. One solution is to claim, after the baby's arrival, that you tried to name the child after her and that it nearly got you laughed out of the maternity ward. Be sure to add, "I just couldn't do that to my child."

PREPARING THE HOUSE FOR BABY'S ARRIVAL (CLEARING OUT THE SPARE CLOSET?)

The new arrival will be your most important guest to date. For the first time, you'll cross the threshold as a family, and it's important to have everything just so, lest baby look down on you. Here are some crucial coming-home elements not to be overlooked.

- Vacuum. Dust-buster. Washing machine. Not for creating a spotless home. For soothing (drowning out?) Baby's colic.

- Lawn stork: To announce to the neighbors your blessed arrival and serve as a convenient landmark for potential baby-snatchers.
- Professionally decorated nursery. If you don't have an elaborate wall mural in place, don't even bother calling yourself a parent.

TAKING A "BABYMOON": ANY EXCUSE TO WADDLE AROUND IN THE SUNSHINE

Some parents opt for one last getaway before we becomes three, and gleeful message boards have dubbed this the babymoon. A babymoon is a lot like a honeymoon but, thanks to the lack of alcohol and your cumbersome body, the sex is so much worse. This in mind, it's better to concentrate on enjoying the trip itself. Of course, now that you're with child, you'll need to tailor your recreational activities accordingly from your pre-pregnant vacations.

For example:

Do: A relaxed beach resort

Don't: Hedonism III

WHAT YOU MAY BE FREAKED OUT ABOUT
Outlaw In-Law?

"My mother-in-law means well, but she wants to live with us shortly after the baby is born. Kill me now."

Although family often offer to pitch in, they sometimes end up being a burden to a recovering mom. Grandparents are especially known for wearing out their welcome while staying over to "help out." But not to worry. Here are some tips that will clear a room of elderly folks quicker than a mild case of E. Coli.

- Block any reruns of *Everybody Loves Raymond* on your television.
- Serve Starbucks or Seattle's Best coffee—any name brand that will offend their thrifty sensibilities.
- Openly mock *Parade* magazine.
- Confiscate all hard candies and mints.
- Ban any sort of clothing or footwear preceded by the word "house."

canine conundrum

"I worry that our pampered pooch will get mad when baby sets up camp. We haven't even told him he won't be the star of our holiday cards anymore."

If you and your dog have shared an unusually close bond, of course there will hurt feelings now that someone new is sharing your bath and suckling at your teat. Fido will see baby as a top-pet threat so it's better to address the problem as early as possible. If you didn't have the forethought to have your pet attend the ultrasound, you can make up for your lapse by bridging the gap as soon as baby arrives. Soon they'll be so close, you won't know where baby ends and dog begins. (Unless baby is being swallowed whole. Then call 911.) Tips for making the transition:

- Make a fun baby rattle fashioned of rawhide and hard dog food.
- Moisturize baby with wet food runoff.
- Confine them both to crib until they "work it out."
- Refer to baby as "new and improved dog."

IS LABOR LOOMING?

Nesting: Discovering the Obsessive-Compulsive in You

If you're in your ninth month and find yourself wiping all contents of the house—floors, counters, guests—with rubbing alcohol, or if you catch yourself organizing your cotton balls by shape, size, and fluffiness, then chances are you've entered a nesting stage. This surge of energy often immediately precipitates labor to allow pregnant women to prepare for their newborn or make one last dash from a life less like hell. Finally noticing those grimy doorjambs or that unacceptable amount of negative ions in the air? Congratulations! You're about to feel some *serious* hurt.

The Low-Down on Luggage

Unless you've mercifully arranged an elective C-section, you never know when the labor bomb is going to drop. In most cases, it will be when your pedicure resembles the talons of an eagle and your hair a disheveled and dirty nest. Thus, it's best to pack a hospital bag beforehand. (If headed to a birthing center, contents still apply but include the dress you'd like to be buried in—just as a precaution, of course!)

Contents of your bag may include:

- A pillow from home so you won't have to share residual skin cells with someone who was actually sick
- Your iPod and favorite downloads so your spouse can drown out your screams
- A billowy, full-length nightgown to shield you from your body's post-birth wreckage

- A list of all contacts, and cell phone or palm pilot, so you can receive congratulations as well as cross off the bastards who don't call
- Your makeup, shampoos, and blow dryer. Trust us, you'll be concentrating on the upper half for a while.

Sample Birth Plan

Here is a template for your baby's big day. Go ahead and fill out your hopes and dreams! Included are physician notes in italics.

LIST OF PEOPLE ALLOWED AT BIRTH

Family or partner_____

Doula_____

Children_____

Lady—you get one damn person, and it's not some voodoo doula. And kids!?! Yeah, go ahead and ruin every subsequent vagina for big brother Johnnie. Thanks, Mom.

ATMOSPHERE

I have a lighting preference.

yes/no

Here's your lighting preference—ON!

I want scented candles.

yes/no

Smell that? Yes, it's total bullshit.

I would like a massage therapist present.

yes/no

> *You need a therapist, period.*

I would like in-room music.

yes/no

> *How about some back-up dancers, too? Get real.*

LABOR AND BIRTH

I would like an epidural.

yes/no

> *Can the staff have one as well? Dealing with you is already incredibly painful.*

If no epidural, I would like to walk around during labor.

yes/no

> *How about doing all of us a big favor and walking to the other hospital? Or nearby spa, where you apparently think you are in the first place.*

I would like to be allowed to labor as long as possible.

yes/no

> *So long as we can leave to eat or smoke, you stay in there until the kid's first birthday.*

I would like baby to have limited fetal monitoring.

yes/no

> *Okay, we'll just use our psychic powers to mind-read how baby is coping.*

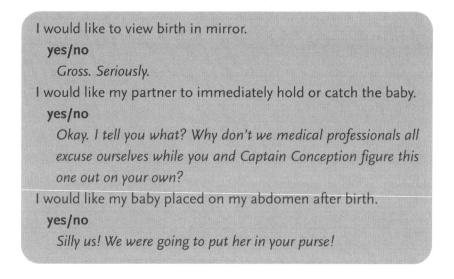

I would like to view birth in mirror.

yes/no

Gross. Seriously.

I would like my partner to immediately hold or catch the baby.

yes/no

Okay. I tell you what? Why don't we medical professionals all excuse ourselves while you and Captain Conception figure this one out on your own?

I would like my baby placed on my abdomen after birth.

yes/no

Silly us! We were going to put her in your purse!

Preparing Your Hospital Birth Plans: Your Dreams/Their Comic Relief

While at the hospital, you'll want to supply the hospital attendants with your birth plan (see previous sample). Make plenty of duplicates. It will be inconvenient to make the staff gather around one copy to make fun of you. To make sure your wishes are realized, remember you get more flies with honey.* In the case of physicians, emblazon it on a gift carton of cigarettes or scroll it around a bottle if liquor. For nurses and techs, panel the inside a box of éclairs or append to scratch lotto. Even though there are bound to be shift changes while you're laboring, it's important to not thrust your birth plan in the face of the new on-duty attendant. To get what you want, a relaxed approach is

---

*But the most flies with a dead body.

best and flattery will get you everywhere. Possible persuasive openers can include:

- "Has anyone told you that you look like McDreamy/Izzie?"
- "I bet a lot of patients wish *you* had gotten them pregnant."
- "Not everyone can carry off that little surgical cap, but it really works on you."
- "Forceps? With you, it feels like fore*play!*"

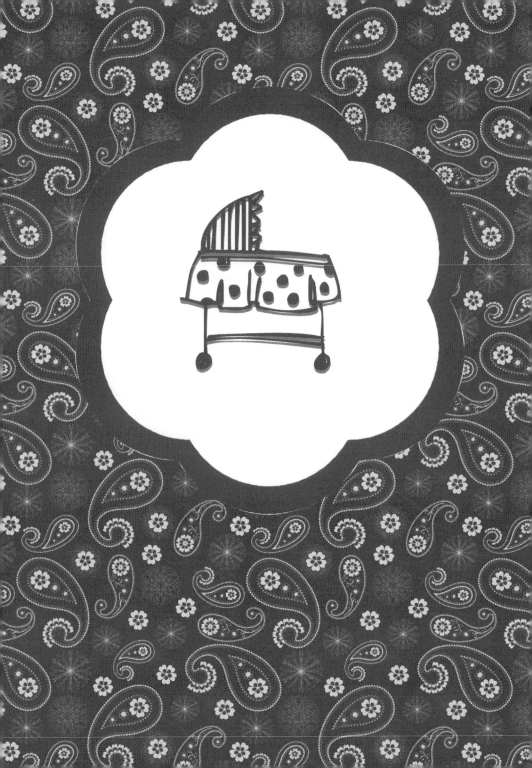

CHAPTER 8

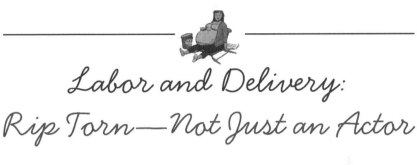

Labor and Delivery: Rip Torn—Not Just an Actor

Bring this book to the hospital. By the time you're in active labor, you'll have little time to review the text, but its size makes it an effective tool for smacking the nearest grating individual. And lo, there will be a host to choose from: your spouse, the one stupid nurse who will mess up or delay something major, and, if birthing off-hours, the bleary-eyed resident physician who will treat you like a medical one-night stand. If you've chosen to forgo an epidural, you can also use the book to bludgeon yourself unconscious. It will be a merciful fate compared to what lies ahead.

WHAT YOU MAY BE FREAKED OUT ABOUT
Uncomfortably Numb

"I'm afraid of the pain. I can barely tolerate a junior Tampax, much less a set of shoulders. Still, I hear epidurals can sometimes cause permanent nerve damage. Is it worth the risk?"

Ironic, since risk-taking is what got you here in the first place. An epidural is no more dangerous than a human being tearing its way out of your backside. You want nerve damage? Watch one of those horrific birthing films of a granola mom who forgoes pain meds. That will wreck your nerves. Sure, the syringe looks painful, but so does an emerging head. Take the damn shot.

Death Becomes Her

"I know it's silly, but I have a fear I might actually die in childbirth! Not to mention the horror of being buried in maternity clothes. Is it possible?"
Sure, if you voted for Taft. Although giving birth is a serious medical procedure, you're no more likely to die than you are at the leeching performed at your compound later. So don't get your pantaloons in a knot. Try to relax and trust the skilled professionals who have done this hundreds of times successfully. Concentrate on the things you can control, like making your own lye and buying baby more war bonds.

Loose Lips Sink Relationships?

"I'm afraid my vagina will change after I have the baby. My husband has never been to the Grand Canyon, and I don't want him to start now. Will he notice the difference during sex?"
He will, but if he ever wants to enter its roomy walls again, he'll lie. Keep in mind, you just passed a human cannonball through that flap. (Think the running of the bulls, but from your bottom.) Above all, be patient with the amount of time needed to feel like yourself again. It could take upwards of six months to return to the tight little package he fell in love with. Note that Kegels

exercising the muscles that make up the pelvic floor, can help during this recovery period. So can exercising the muscles of your jaw.

As Labor Loses All Appeal

Stage 1: Dilation to 3 cm. *I can do this.*
Stage 2: Dilation to 7 cm. *Wow. This really hurts.*
Stage 3: Dilation to 10 cm. *There is no God.*

The First cut Is the Deepest

"My doctor says circumcision is mainly a cosmetic concern. Is skin really in?"
What are a few moments of forgotten pain to avoid years of women talking about him over cocktails? And that doesn't include being subjected to the word "thingy." No man wants to spend the rest of his life looking down at a windsock. Besides, having a foreskin involves extra care in cleaning—or pulling back a flap. A man can't even bother vacuuming under the couch, much less his penis. Need more proof? Go look in your partner's car/office/gym locker and apply that to his genitals. Do you really want discarded fast food wrappers and empty Red Bull cans littering your son's nethers? We didn't think so.

A Guide for the coach: Up to Bat in the Field of Screams

"Okay, I got her into this mess. How can I best help my spouse during labor?"
Although labor is difficult endure, having to watch your partner writhing in pain isn't exactly easy. Still, even on its worst day, it

does beat being torn in half. Here is what your laboring partner would tell you if she could stop the stream of expletives for even a moment.

- "Shut up. Whatever you say will just be plain wrong."
- "Say something. Don't just sit there while I writhe in pain."
- "Get involved. Take charge so I don't have to."
- "Stay out of it. You're just going to muck everything up."

Now that you have clear instructions on how to be effective as a coach, you can expect similar consistency when it comes to her expectations of you as a father. Welcome to eighteen-plus years of failing miserably.

STAGE ONE: WHEN YOU REALIZE THERE'S NO EASY WAY OUT

Phase One: Early Pain

This is the stage of labor in which you foolishly overestimate your ability to survive childbirth. Indicators include being able to hold a conversation without becoming violent, and tolerating mindless sitcoms.

DAD'S TO-DO:
Play cervical concierge: offer pillows, fetch ice, or update her magazine rotation.

Phase Two: Active Pain

This stage is shorter than the last but makes up for it in intensity and sheer regret. If you've opted to not have an epidural, you'll start to realize that you have been deluded and arrogant throughout the pregnancy and this is nature's way of taking you down, bitch. With an epidural, you'll happily continue chomping ice chips and reading gossip rags. Natural birth? Suckers!

DAD'S TO-DO:
If in pain, massage her back (it will be harder for her to smack you) and act as medical go-between so she doesn't have to expend extra energy threatening personnel directly.

Phase Three: Advanced Pain

For non-epidural goers, this stage can be best described as demonic possession. You will recoil at human touch except in the case of inflicting pain on others. You'll invent new curses and be convinced that God has no mercy. But even the epidural bunch doesn't get off easy. In a horrible turn of events, you'll be jerked from that Novocain bliss to push, allowing you to dive in and experience labor as raw as if you birthed in a cave. All the while, you'll mentally kick yourself for not preparing a will and having settled for that useless asshole who's in the corner rocking and shaking uncontrollably. Happy birthday.

DAD'S TO-DO:
Offer a new car and Tiffany diamonds, and stay out of arm's reach.

STAGE TWO "I'M COMING OUT AND YOU'RE GOING DOWN"

Now that you've reached the active stage of labor, which involves pushing the baby—and, in some cases, various individuals—you may find yourself in one of two positions—supine and gutted like a fish or upright and splayed like a pornographic fiddler crab. Either way, you can take solace. The vaginal delivery group can tout their scar-free abdomens, while C-section veterans can make the proud claim that they didn't crap the table. In fact, these opposing ends of the birth spectrum are the perfect introduction to the mutually supportive community that is Camp Mom. (By the way, breast is best and anything less is child abuse.)

See?

RECOVERING AFTER STARING INTO THE MOUTH OF HELL

You've just undergone a major medical procedure, so it's natural that throngs of people should visit while your placenta is still attached. Never mind the impaired vision from the vein that burst in your eye mid-push—it's hostess time! If you're lucky, you might even be able to whip out your boob in front of your father-in-law or have your perineum stitched in that viewing auditorium once known as your hospital room. The good news is, you can be lying in a pool of your own blood and no one will care. You've done a fine job of being the vessel for your in-laws' namesake. Now scram, flabby. It's all about the baby now.

Extended Hospital Stays: Fully Insured? Stay as Long as You Like!

If you underwent a C-section, you may have to stay at the hospital for up to a week. According to the nursing staff, there is no more perfect time for you to start intensive care of your newborn than the immediate hours after abdominal surgery. Most hospitals will claim to have prenatal nursery care to allow you to occasionally rest, but they're only for the truly negligent mothers. For the most part, the message is abundantly clear: take some Vicodin and get to work. You've got a baby to raise, and we have a break to take. A shower, you ask? This isn't Canyon Ranch, lady. How else will you learn to diaper your fragile infant while grasping a hospital bed rail, trembling in pain? What do you think we're here for? To medically assist you and care for you?

Besides, someone has to pay for that less-than-stellar GPA that kept them from med school, and it might as well be you, princess.

Two's a crowd

"I decided to share a room with my baby after the delivery, but I'm finding it exhausting. She keeps crying and, well, acting like a baby. Am I already failing as a mom?"

Relax. You did something that Hercules could not have accomplished. (That's because Hercules doesn't have a vagina or your poor judgment.) You and baby may have to take it slow and get to know one another. You wouldn't move in right away with some weirdo from Craigslist. Is this baby any less of a stranger?

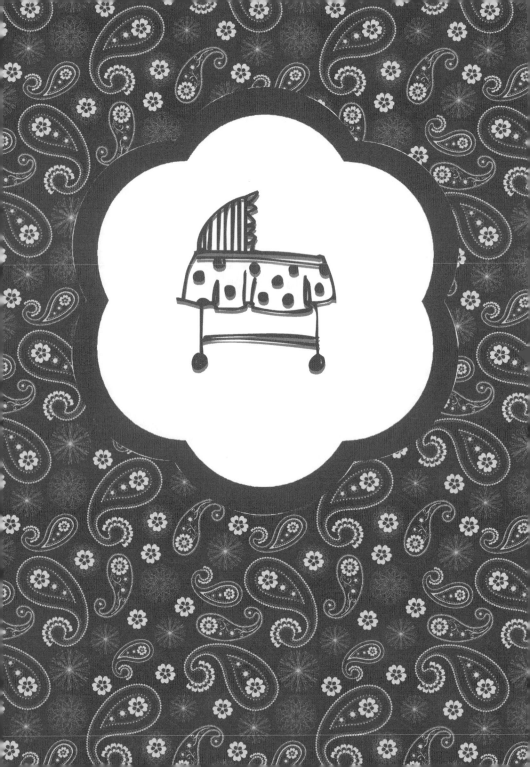

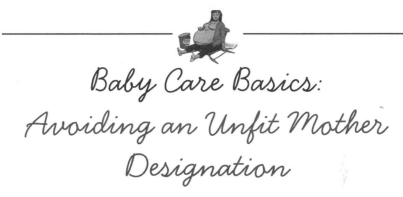

CHAPTER 9

Baby Care Basics: Avoiding an Unfit Mother Designation

DIAPER HOW-TO: WHICH ELMO GOES IN THE FRONT??

You're likely stocked up with tiny newborn diapers—and you'll waste almost half when baby immediately outgrows the supply. These are not your mother's diapers (which are bigger and sold in a different aisle). Unless they're cloth*, not only are they easily disposed of, they often bear the faces of popular characters. (Today's: Dora the Explorer or Winnie-the-Pooh; yesterday's: Jack Benny and Spiro Agnew.) They also come in a fitted, hourglass shape, a little engineering detail that only took thirty or so years to iron out. Luckily, people aren't as dumb now as they were back then (*I Love Lucy*: case in point) and you, new parent, reap the rewards. Between the hours of convenient absorption and comfort fit, diaper-changing is practically becoming an optional daily duty. Negligent parents: one; court-appointed monitors: zero.

---

* Idiot.

changing for the Better

THE BOTTOM LINE IN BOTTOM CARE: HOW TO HANDLE HANDLING EXCREMENT

Lay baby on changer. Try amusing baby with silly faces or singsong conversations about your latest problems. Remember, baby doesn't understand the words, just the tone. For example, "Mommy is sleeping on the couch because Daddy-Waddy doesn't want to touch her anymore. *No, he doesn't...*"

For newborns, be sure to use sensitive-care wet wipes. Save your bathroom staple of "rough and cheap" for the in-laws who overstay their welcome.

Lotions are okay, but avoid the powder. Baby might breathe into lungs and end up looking like you did at The China Club circa 1989.

Waste Management

"I know disposable diapers are easiest, but are they the best choice? See, I'm one of those moms for whom convenience is evil."

Good question. As far back as anyone cares, parents have had to decide how to contain baby's waste (neighbor's garbage?). But you, modern mom (and occasional trespasser), you won't have to go to such extremes to keep baby's bottom in top form. What's right will depend a lot on convenience versus environmental concerns. Here's what to consider when it comes to the great diaper debate.

DISPOSABLE DIAPERS: MAN, THESE THINGS ROCK.

For the mom who has any sort of life, these are the sole option. If you can barely handle grass stains in your laundry, let alone fecal matter, you'll find any other alternative laughable at best. The only downside is that today's diapers are so absorbent, they might lead to infrequent changes.* There's also the landfill issue to consider, which is easily resolved since it's in the landfill, and thus not your problem anymore. Don't let those environmental worrywarts get to you. You want an inconvenient truth? Plastic is awesome. Besides, *you'll* be hazardous waste long before those Huggies have a stranglehold on the planet. *But the children*, some green parent might contest. By the time of your death, you'll have fractured your relationship to the point that a gaping ozone will be the final finger those little ingrates deserve.

Hey, and they have cute little animals on them, too!

CLOTH DIAPERS: JUST AS SOON AS I START MAKING MY OWN CLOTHES

If you want to avoid plastic and convenience altogether, cloth diapers are for you. You might buy the environment a little more time, but it will be shaved off your own life as you wrestle that little squirmer into an ill-fitting napkin. To avoid leaks, you'll still need additional waterproof pants, which seem a lot like, well, diapers. And for fewer occurrences of rash, you'll also have fewer occurrences of a social life, as cloth diapers hold you hostage to the nearest changing area—God forbid baby takes a tiny wee. While you're at it, why not trade in your washing machine for a washboard and give up your right to vote? Let's potty like it's 1899!

---

*This is a downside?

CLEAN IT UP

Unless your little one is spending his days in the coal mines*, bathing is one of the baby-care basics where you can afford flexibility. Even with intermittent bathing, your infant may still protest at tub time. You can help ease her anxieties with these simple waterproof rules:

- A separate cloth should be used for bathing baby's diaper area. Baby doesn't want to use an ass rag on his face any more than you do.
- If baby expresses anxiety during bathing process, comfort with a steady hold and reassuring words like, "I've seen CPR on *Baywatch* thousands of times."
- After bathing baby, dry and wrap in towel—*then* shampoo and rinse her hair. It will keep baby warm and more content throughout process.**

Bathing Prep

You'll need more than a rubber duckie. You won't be able to leave baby's side for a moment, no matter how buoyant his blubber makes him seem. This in mind, it's crucial to have every supply in arm's reach. Your list for lathering up:

SOFT TERRYCLOTH RAG:

Wash gently with a cotton cloth and resist the temptation to exfoliate baby. It might take a few hours off his rapidly aging skin, but for that pink, supple hide, only the gentle touch of a baby-soft cloth will do. (Note: anti-aging regimen is best begun

---

*Exception for babies from Kentucky or West Virginia which are often born in coal mines
**An actual piece of advice. We thought you'd like to get *something* useful out of this book.

at age four when the stress of Gymboree and Mommy and Daddy's fighting begins to show on preschool skin.)

TEAR-FREE SOAP AND SHAMPOO:
Use products specifically formulated for infants and avoid anything boasting "new and improved strength" or "that stuff that makes up Comet" in the list of ingredients.

DRYING TOWEL:
With a hood and something hilarious like a frog, duck, or sheep.*
Non-hooded is acceptable; non-hilarious is not.

DIAPER BALM:
Anything but the "salve" grandma mixed up for you.

The Gross Stump that Will Eventually Become a Cute Belly Button

It's as pleasant as it sounds. The umbilical is the last remaining connection between the two of you—sort of like baby is to your relationship with your husband. Within the first month, it will turn black, wither, and fall away (not unlike your significant other's heart). To help the healing, apply alcohol. Ditto for baby's umbilical.

Audio: The Forgotten Hole

As should go for most orifices, never stick anything smaller than a penis in your ear—and you better be damn drunk when that

---

*Avoid real ducks. Except in the case of fluffy down comforters or delicious pâtés.

happens. Outer-ear cleaning should be more than enough for your little one. (Also, never penetrate the ear canal. If it helps, think of Q-Tips as cotton-encased spears.) Wax buildup is normal in the ear unless, say, you could construct a celebrity likeness from the excess. If that's the case, consult your physician or the curator of Madame Tussaud's.

HOLDING YOUR BABY: NOT BY THE NAPE

Wrap It Up

Some babies love the feel of swaddling, of a soothing arm constraint that reminds them of the tight fit of the womb. Others dislike the inability to do frivolous things like shield their eyes from the blinding sunlight or fend off disgruntled pets.

If you have a baby who prefers the straitjacket, take heart. Swaddling is as simple as a making a spicy morning meal. Just wrap baby as you would a delicious breakfast burrito. Bundle tightly—you wouldn't want the stuff to fall out of the bottom, would you? (Stuff = baby.)

Picking Baby Up

In order not to startle baby, it's important to let him or her know you're about to pick them up. Approach using eye contact along with these possible openers.

BABY PICK-UP LINES:

- "You have fewer folds than most babies. And I'm not just saying that."

- "Your hand-eye coordination rivals that of a myopic first grader."
- "That scent of baby lotion and strained prunes is intoxicating."
- "I love the way your hair wisps in the wind like Woodstock from *Peanuts*."

BABY AS A FASHION STATEMENT

This can be one of the surprisingly frustrating rites of newborn care. Dressing and undressing baby, you'll soon discover that she is ridiculously out of shape. You've waited nine months to clothe this child, and it's painfully apparent she did nothing during the gestational period besides parasitic snacking, along with treating your bladder like a couch. Wrestling with her oversized head, floppy sausage-like arms, and generally shapeless form, you may even start to feel like Star Jones' stylist. Try not to be critical, at least in baby's presence. You have to work with what you've got,

The Irreverent Onesie

YOU'RE COOL. WE GET IT...

Now please stop. By the time you are reading these words, we can only hope the trend is over. But it won't be. *Why?* you ask. Because every nine months or so, another crop of newbies comes along and says "Baby expresses an adult sentiment? It can't be! I must purchase two...no, make that ten!" Aren't you unique, hip, and funny? No, no, and no. Take that and iron it on a onesie.

Worst offenders:

"Daddy's Little Princess": Really? The royal family resides in Oklahoma? Face it. The closest you're going to come to nobility is the Dairy Queen uniform that awaits you.

"Here comes trouble!": Here comes unoriginality. I'm going to guess your parents aren't members of the Writer's Guild.

"Grandma says I can!": Grandma also hides in the hamper every time the UPS man comes to the door, convinced he's with the Gestapo. Better choose a better advocate, kid.

so here are some immediate camouflaging techniques that will help hide baby's multitude of sins.

- Concentrate on close-up pics of baby's face. This is often practiced by new parents. Now you know why.
- Skim a pound of baby-announcement weight. The lies have to start sometime.
- High chairs and swings are great visual obstructions to hide baby's ample hip spread.
- Hang out with fatter babies. (Diabetic moms are a wonderful resource of oversized infants!)

Once your baby finally hits a decent goal weight, clothes can be a matter of practicality (for warmth or airy comfort) or a billboard of your personal agendas ("God planned me, and my mommy votes.") Above all, your focus should be safety and ease of wear, so it's best to veer from that asbestos-lined jumper or Spandex onesie even if it does hug baby in all the right places.

Today, children's clothing options are endless. Some designers offer mother/daughter sets, allowing mom to look infantile or baby to look like a slut, while dad-and-son combos bring out the IT guy in most anyone.

RARE DISORDERS
Postpartum Entrepreneurial Syndrome

There's something about postpartum hormones that brings out the madcap inventor in any mom. Maybe it's all that time at home alone or the realization that you can't get by on looks alone now, not to mention your mass introduction to some of the world's most poorly made products. Whatever the case, there isn't a new mother out there who hasn't fondled a BeDazzler while imagining the possibilities. Some have even gone so far as looking up on the Internet how to obtain a patent (although most get sidetracked by checking in on their mommyblog). Full of blind optimism (thanks to upping dosage) she's sure that her camo "Baby Supports the Troops" onesie is going to change the face of QVC.* As nature intends, the postnatal hormones are eventually released from the body along with the dreams of becoming the next Julie Aigner-Clark** (the mother who created the Baby Einstein empire). Soon enough, the rhinestones fall away (possibly in baby's trachea) and somewhere a cold wind whips though an empty aisle at Hobby Lobby.

---

*Impossible to change the face of QVC. Too much Botox. On a side note, QVC stands for Quit inVenting Crap. Okay, it's a stretch. Oh yeah. You're a mom now... Actually, this is a perfectly fine joke. You're just too tired/out of touch with other adults to get it.

**It is a little-known fact that Julie Aigner-Clark is not a mother at all, but a lifelike, digitally-enhanced image created by Disney and the creative whizzes at Pixar.

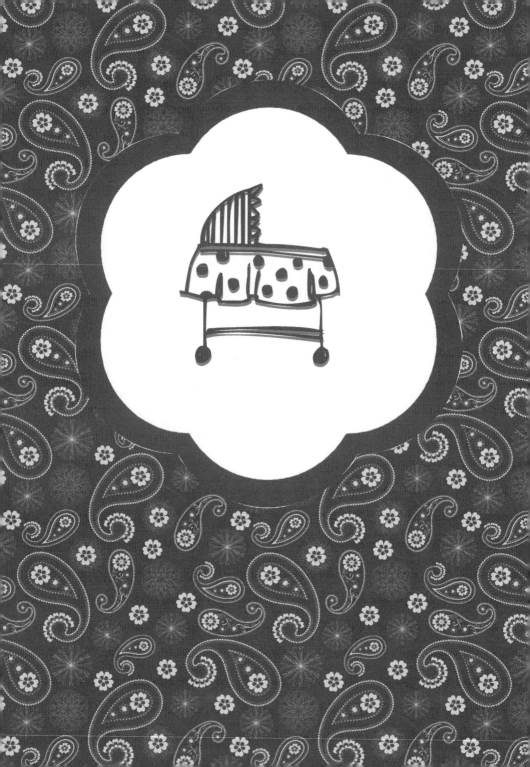

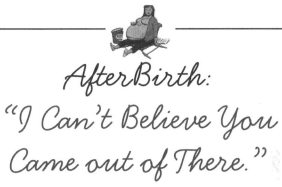

CHAPTER 10

AfterBirth:
"I Can't Believe You
Came out of There."

You finally have that little rascal in your arms, and she's looking less like Ed Asner every day. You, on the other hand, are another story. With a deflated gut, bags under your eyes and newly thinning hair, you look less like a mother and more like a Founding Father. If nursing, your breasts have likely monopolized most of the space between your collarbone and that marshlike landscape once known as your stomach. You may also feel a little mentally unstable, vacillating between sheer elation and stay-at-home mom despair. Luckily, all it takes is a long, sweet gaze at that tiny miracle to know one thing for certain.

You did this to me.

This could very well be the onset of the baby blues, which occurs sometime between arriving home and the onslaught of every jerk with a casserole recipe showing up.

WHAT YOU MAY BE FREAKED OUT ABOUT
Bond Girl

"My preemie baby girl had to spend time in the ICU. It took me a week to realize that 'I see you' wasn't a cute name for the viewing window of the maternity ward. In any case, will it hinder my bonding with her?"

If she didn't get a chance to bond with you, don't worry your emotionally distant head about it. She'll think you're a total bitch by her eleventh birthday anyway. Recent studies show most of the previous findings on the need for initial bonding have proved baseless. Just look to all the healthy children raised by non-biological parents. (Just avoid peeking too far ahead into their drug-addled and promiscuous teen years.) Your baby doesn't remember a thing from those early hours. Being cuddled by a gorilla won't make her hanker for bananas. But if she didn't bond with her *father*, later on, she'll most certainly hanker for anything attached to a much-older penis. On that, the research is irrefutable.

Post-Baby Carnage

"I know I should be easier on myself about just having had a baby, but I can't help but feel my husband can't be attracted to my postpartum body. I feel like three deflated balloons on a couple of tree trunks. Sexy, right?"

Almost every woman fears her husband finds her less attractive post-birth. And in this case, they're right. Face it, you're no Heidi Klum now, so you might as well do the best you can with that car wreck you call a physique. There are ways to entice him even in those unrecognizable first weeks after baby. Creative coupling games can include:

- "Let's Talk About Your Hot Friend"
- "From Behind…Every Time"
- "Your Mouth Didn't Get Fat…"

Baby Blues: Beyond Turquoise, Navy, and Cobalt
Wait, this still sucks…

This may be your continued feeling about bringing home what is turning out to be eight pounds of lame. You may feel betrayed that your baby, far from mugging like the babies on commercials, isn't giving 100 percent or at least meeting you halfway. You have to change his diaper—the least he can do is iron out a few of those wrinkles and fake a smile occasionally. Even though you may be feeling impatient, it's normal for baby to take a few months to pull it together. In the meantime, you can pretend he's one of those purse Chihuahuas that are all the rage.

But if a bedimpled smile and sparkling eyes don't emerge, you may have to come to terms with having a plain baby (PB) or, worse, an unattractive baby (UB). Determining baby's level of appeal is crucial. Since you're somewhat invested in this tyke and can't possibly be objective, how do you know if you've got a Jessica Simpson on your hands, or alternatively, an Ashlee Simpson? Gorgeous babies are often greeted with business cards and television pilots. Plain babies are often greeted with noncommittal phrases like "Isn't she something!" or "What a sweetheart." Meanwhile, unattractive babies are even more generalized. ("Nice stroller!" or "Do you know what time it is?")

If a less-than-good-looking baby isn't what is prolonging your sadness, you could be suffering from postpartum depression, a serious condition that, when handled correctly, can lead to high-profile interviews and lucrative book deals. In most cases, medication is necessary, and—let's face it—just fun. While other "level" moms will have to contend with the ups and downs of babyhood, you'll be the princess of the prescription pad, blissfully unaware of all that you've lost. Besides, mental illness is considered very chic and exotic in certain circles. Play your cards right and you'll be snapping Larry King's suspenders in no time.

YOU HAVE TO LEAVE THE HOUSE
Mommy's Baggage

Remember when you were able to jet out the door with a set of keys and a medium-sized purse? Those days are long gone. From now on, your public self will resemble something like a wayward Sherpa who mistook Toys "R" Us for Patagonia. Here's what consists of your new mother "load."

Diaper Bag

Large and cumbersome, it's going to be right by your side for the next couple of years. But enough about baby. The bag you carry will need to be stocked and reviewed daily to ensure you can parent on the go. Here are the essentials:

AS MANY EXTRA DIAPERS AS YOU CAN CARRY:
If you're wearing white, take a box. Baby won't be satisfied until he's made a mural on your Donna Karan.

MOIST TOWELETTES:
For baby's bottom and mother's frequent crying jags.

CHANGE OF CLOTHES:
In case your baby is not as dressed up as surrounding babies.

BAGGIES:
For carrying and disposing of baby's dirty diapers so you can avoid having to ask horrified shop owners, "Can I throw this away in here?"

LIQUID LUNCH:
Unless you're boobing it, baby needs his mix fix.

Bad Rides

If this is your second child or you live more than five miles from your city's downtown, you're going to end up an owner of a utility vehicle. It isn't a choice; it is your destiny. For women, this means more space to store all those shopping bags and plenty of elbow room for the kids. For men, it means giving away their prized Porsche, and locking their penis away in the glove box. You can talk all day about the swivel seats and dual video monitors, but face it: you are so lame now. Like all things that we try to pretend don't suck, there's always someone who has it a little worse than you. (This is the urban-planning theory on which suburbs were founded.) Here is the SUV food chain:

LAND ROVER/HUMMER/ALL-TERRAIN VEHICLE
The person who owns one of these has a vehicle for children but is so far in denial that you may find their offspring accidentally

embedded in the grill. Fathers especially will try to justify the purchase as cool or masculine given the size and expense. *It could be for hauling my gear on camping trips or tearing up the terrain on my next mountain adventure*, they tell themselves. My dear misled man. The only adventure you'll be taking is at Babies "R" Us, and your "gear" will consist of whatever your wife allows. So go ahead and hang your hopes—and your testicles—from the rearview mirror. But don't worry. It's nothing a fifty-two-inch television and a mistress won't fix. (Both easily stored with all that additional cargo room!)

LUXURY SUV

You know you're no longer cool, but you are going down fighting anyway. You're the person driving with a latte in one hand and tiny phone in the other*, steering with your elbow while complaining loudly about the latest slight by your poolhand/nanny/gardener.** (Meanwhile, they stare out the passenger windows, helpless to both your tirade and immigration laws.) *But Nelly drives an Escalade!* you protest. *I'm still cool, right?* Nelly isn't sporting a "Mother of an Honor Student" sticker on the back. Nelly's got a wet bar and is kickin' it old school; not Wet Wipes, kickin' it preschool.

SUBURBAN

You stopped trying a long time ago. With your sensible short haircut and high-waisted jeans, you're the captain of the captain's

---

*Or worse, Bluetooth ear set. You may be safer driving, but you're so annoying; is that in anyone's best interest?

**Unless your SUV is a used, certified pre-owned. Then you're complaining about the richer bitch next door, knowing full well you'll never quite measure up.

chair. That doesn't mean you're afraid to throw caution to the wind. Along with occasionally substituting margarine for butter, you've been know to "go Mrs. Dash" all over that casserole. Good times. Meanwhile, the real dash should be from that manicured lawn you call a life. Plus, you worship at the altar of Rachael Ray. You TiVoed her show, didn't you? Sorry, but there's just nothing we can do to help you.

Baby Sounds Like a Screech Owl:
Please Translate

So how do you know when baby is really in need versus just being a neonatal narcissist? Here is a crib sheet to help you decipher the crying game.

"MAYBE YOU SHOULD ENROLL IN A BABY CLASS" CRY
Short and low-pitched, this is baby's way of undermining your confidence and expressing his or her doubt about your parental abilities. It is generally preceded by baby's attempt to flag down strangers (often mistaken as random arm flailing) or desperate efforts to attract attention through aggressive shaking of rattles or toys. Innocent banging on the table or S.O.S. signal? You can never be sure.

"I HATE WHAT YOU'RE WATCHING" CRY
This is baby's plea for you to turn off *The Bachelor* or the latest loud, insipid nighttime game show. Also known as the "Where's Charlie Rose?" wail or the "De Niro's on *Inside the Actor's Studio*" plea.

"SERIOUSLY, AM I WITH THE TWO OF YOU FOR EIGHTEEN YEARS?" CRY

This whiny, high-pitched moan is baby's final realization that there will be no celebrity adoption. Surveying his less-than-stellar surroundings, baby can't help but realize a future with you will be limited. There will be no first-class flights or humanitarian visits to Africa. And damned if there will be a trust fund, unless trusting in the Lord counts. And it doesn't.

"I HATE YOUR TASTE IN NURSERY DÉCOR" CRY

There's nothing more soothing to a baby than feeling like he's living inside a cartoon cell. Who wouldn't want to romp amongst Disney's woodland creatures that in real life would eviscerate baby or, at best, leave a mess of hoof imprints about his tiny body? Notice this is a weaker cry with a lower pitch, possibly because he can't catch enough air in his lungs while choking on the still-fresh fumes of the eerie woodland mural that haunts his dreams. Please paint over those bastardized images your art-school-dropout cousin created on your wall and prevent Walt Disney from ever wanting to reattach his head.

WHAT YOU MAY BE FREAKED OUT ABOUT
Newborn Paranoia

"I love being a mother, but I live in fear that my baby will stop breathing. Am I crazy? Oh, can you pass me that Rid? If I delouse our dog's hair strand by strand, nothing bad will happen."

Crazy? No, not if you know where we live. You're simply a bit neurotic, and it's nothing that intensive therapy or monitored medication won't cure. The truth is, all babies exhibit erratic breathing patterns. This is how baby jacks with you. You try staring at a mobile all day and see if you don't come up with some twisted head games. Other ways baby messes with you: crying at all hours, supposedly because he's hungry, and repeatedly dropping things. Don't be fooled. He may lack the language ability to express it but, watching you slave to his beck and call, he can't help but think, *What a jerk*. Besides, who's wiping whose ass?

WHERE'S THE ME IN MOMMY?
Finding Your Body Again

Congratulations—once more! You're now the *least* hot woman at the gym. (Unless you work out at an all-women's gym or twenty-four-hour fitness center where the clientele is decidedly less attractive as a whole.) If you work out at a chic coed facility that serves smoothies, never fear. Half the members are gay men anyway. Still, it's not unreasonable to freeze your membership until you're cute enough to work out there. It's the right thing to do.

See Ya, Soccer Moms

"My maternity leave is winding down, and although I love my baby, I miss the respect I get from being legitimately employed—you don't get a W-2 from being a mommy! Ha! What can I do to ensure an easy transition back to the real world?"

Well, Little Miss Ambition…should have thought about that when you were picking away at that glass ceiling. Inevitably, the shards have to fall somewhere, and it looks like baby's got a bull's-eye on her bald, soon-to-be-abandoned pate. Not to say you should have any guilt. Six or more figures can buy you loads of childhood therapy for attachment issues. *Of course, we're joking!* Everyone knows that the working mom versus stay-at-home mom debate is just another issue where women agree to disagree. Each woman must make the choice that works for her family. (Just ask any of those worthless bitches wasting their MBAs at Gymboree!) At home or at work, the important thing is to let your child know she is loved. Here are some tips to make Mommy's "bye-bye" a little easier.

- Load up on tons of material goods to make up for absence. Remember, nothing says love like a mini-Cadillac Escalade or Bratz doll.
- Provide the best almost-English-proficient care a parent can hire (see Chapter 11).
- Record songs sung by you for little one to enjoy. Insist nanny lip-sync for full effect.
- Have your assistant send baby-loving emails every hour.
- Teleconference a story.

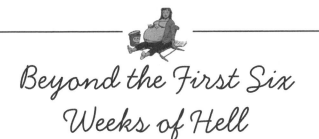

Beyond the First Six Weeks of Hell

WHO WILL BABY LOVE MORE THAN YOU?

Sitters or nannies aren't only for working moms. At some point, parents will want to go out alone and will have to trust someone else to care for their most precious possession. And depending on where you live, family isn't always an option.

Unlike older children, six-week-old Sammy can't tell you if the babysitter has been drinking all the cough syrup, so research and diligence are of the utmost importance. In ancient times, one had to perform a criminal background check, but today's sitter does it for you. It's called MySpace and/or Facebook. Who needs references when you can read your potential caretaker's poem about failing calculus or attending her latest rainbow lipstick party? Inexplicably ignoring the privacy mode, today's young person allows you a wonderful gateway into the youth culture that may or may not try on your jewelry (or your husband) when you're out of the house. If you're lucky enough to find a young person immune to Internet broodings or an older, single lover of cats, then you're ready to bestow upon them the responsibility of a lifetime: making sure that nothing gets spilled on your couch. Oh, and that baby is safe and happy.

Interviewing a Potential Mistress, Uh, Sitter

QUESTIONS TO ASK YOUR PROSPECTIVE CHILDCARE PROVIDER:

Recreation wise, how do you see yourself spending the day as a caregiver?

Good answer: "Based on your baby's age and developmental level..."

Bad answer: "Based on the size of your pool and liquor cabinet..."

Who was your last employer and why did you leave that position?

Good answer: "The Johnson family. They and their six children moved out of the country, although they offered to take me with them."

Bad answer: "Hooters. Which reminds me, those bastards still have my check."

What do you think an average schedule would be?

Good answer: "Once baby wakes, feeding, then a bath followed by requisite stories and interactive play. By the way, I'm a stickler for routine..."

Bad answer: "Wake up around eleven. Go back to my own house. On the way, hit that Mexican fast-food joint for a breakfast taco followed by an Advil/Pepto chaser...Oh. You're talking about with the baby?"

What do you think a baby needs most?

Good answer: "Lots of attention and stimulation."

Bad answer: "Oxygen. That's what the autopsy said."

How would you handle disciplinary issues?

Good answer: "Consistency is key…"

Bad answer: "My boyfriend makes an extra set of keys…and we have a safety word."

Do you have experience with CPR training?

Good answer: "I was certified five years ago and take a refresher course each year for fun."

Bad answer: "Yes. They performed it on me when I went unconscious at the Phi Kappa frat mixer last month. At least that's what the house brothers told me they were doing."

Sit-Sense

Without a single word, you can learn a lot from first impressions, so listen to your gut instinct. For example:
- Did she present her résumé from a neat folder or tote?
- Did she present her résumé from the inked palate of her inner arm?
- Did she speak fluent English?
- Did she start her sentences with "Me" followed by any array of verbs?

AT YOUR PLACE

The Au Pair

Depending on what generation you're from, an au pair may make you think of airborne umbrellas or violent shaking. In any case, an au pair is generally a foreigner who wants to visit the United States for a year but has to care for your child-in-residence to do it. Most are young, educated individuals from countries like England and Australia whose delightful accents will distract you from the fact they just want you to go to sleep so they can "meet all the beautiful American guys they see on the telly." To this end, kindly direct your in-house foreign horny to the nearest sports bar and gleefully watch the American dream die. Once she realizes the fruited dating plains are about as barren as her new country's economy, she'll resume her rightful place in your laundry room and/or kitchen. Just 364 more days to go, mate!

The Manny

Who says a man can't give the same care and attentiveness as a woman? Many families are starting to hire young men as sitters and find they are especially helpful in caring for young boys who might enjoy watching hours of *SportsCenter*, in addition to offering girls the math edge a female caregiver could never provide. So yes, go ahead and spring for XY tutelage. Just make sure he understands the difference between Wii and wee.

MEET THE PARENTS
When the Grandparents care for Baby

This is a subset of sitter that is a breed all its own. Your first instinct will be to let your guard down, since babies are no mystery to the senior set. They raised you, right? "That's your first mistake, Toots," Grandpa himself might say, if he wasn't outside defecating in the neighbor's yard. Far from being prepared, elderly sitters give you childcare that is a wondrous mix of dementia and borderline witchcraft. There are different types of grandparents out there, though, and it's important to know into which category your parents or in-laws fall and whether or not they can get up.

Types of Elderly Caregivers:

BITTER OLD BASTARDS
"Back in my day..."

Enough said. Check their pockets for mummified candy and lozenges and trade dinner out for a couple of quick drinks—preferably on your porch or in the lobby of your apartment building.

THE SASSY SENIOR
Spry and assured in their golf attire and T-shirt jumper sets, it's tempting to be lured into a state of complacency. Sure, Grandma may have email, but she keeps forwarding those hoaxes, doesn't she? Don't let all their *Dateline*-acquired knowledge fool you. Keep this pair's sitting duties close to home. They'll plead for an overnighter at their house, but invariably, your baby will end up

eating his weight in Plavix or wedged in the gears of their Sleep Number bed. Like the subject line of so many of their email forwards: *Beware!*

More Grandparent Dilemmas

"We want to keep baby on a consistent schedule and we worry about the visiting grandparents spoiling her and putting us back at square one. Plus, we can't stand 60 Minutes."

Grandparents are a wonderful resource—if you exist on a steady diet of damaged fruit and off-brand soda. Like most new parents with loving relatives, you're going to have your hands full as this elderly duo tries to muscle (albeit deteriorating muscle) their way into you and your spouse's care-giving cocoon. Grandpa may mean well, but it can be hard to convince the previous generation that an old war grenade (inactive or not) or a necklace of Japanese teeth aren't appropriate toys. If they live close by, a one-on-one talk should help make the boundaries clear. (And if not, you can always change your phone number and switch out one digit of your house address, leaving them forever stranded and mystified.) But if they only make the occasional appearances, having baby wake at 4 a.m. to avoid being a "lazybones" or giving him rich, buttermilk baths will only reinforce the bond between you and your child with the one thing that brings anyone closer—hating the same people.

DAY CARE: SO YOU MARRIED POOR...

It's a safe bet there aren't any inherited stock shares in your little guy's future. Enter group day care, the more affordable back-to-work option that will make you question your decision to ever procreate with your college T.A. Because this child-care option is run by a group of individuals, there's no crisis if one goes into rehab or gets sent to jail. (Depending on your program's hiring standards, the combined I.Q. points of the remaining employees could dip to the level of that of an extremely astute seeing-eye dog.) And speaking of illness, you'll get an immune-system workout from a host of debilitating bugs courtesy of those little virus incubators—infectious strains a terrorist could only dream about. Who needs germ warfare when you can just accidentally drink from the same sippie?

Playing Day care Detective

Centers range from top-notch (employees with no criminal records and mastery of basic hygiene skills) to the worst (combined childcare/gator farm). Here is the least you should expect from your child-care center.

ACCREDITATION:
Most states cover the bare-bones operational requirements— but not if your day care runs *Dora* on a loop while they while they "take some 'me' time."

WELL-TRAINED EMPLOYEES:
The head teacher should have more than just a head. Experience working at places like Chuck E. Cheese is preferred, while the rest of the staff should have a background in infant care beyond just having spotted one at a mall.

NON-CONTAGIOUS STAFF:
Ask if the child-care workers have been vetted by a doctor and have all required shots. If a staffer approaches you with yellow eyes or solicits your urine, look elsewhere.

PLENTY OF EYES ON BABY:
The number of staffers depends on the size of your day care but no one should be juggling more than three kids. In other words…the maximum amount of people you would have allowed in your bed back when you were single.

SIZE—SOMETHING BETWEEN A CUBICLE AND AN AIRPORT TERMINAL:
You don't want stadium day care, nor do you want to leave your kid in something the size of your first apartment. If your child has to take a moving sidewalk to class or alternatively keeps choking on the hair of the child next to them, search for a middle ground.

KIDDIES CORRALLED—BY AGE:
You don't want a bunch of sullen teens loitering around and depressing your infant.

WARM AND FUZZY VIBE:
If cries are met with, "Oh, grow up!" and "I just changed you three hours ago!" exercise caution.

A WELL-MAINTAINED AND PROFESSIONAL FACILITY:
Beware if your in-home child-care director gives you a tour of the laundry/reading room.

POSTPARTUM SOCIALIZING: NETWORKING WITH OTHER MOMS

The first few weeks with a newborn can be an isolating experience. Luckily, the Internet is a café of new companions where bad hair or baby weight is irrelevant, but harsh criticism and a sense of superiority are essential. (If you don't know how to photo-share online, please don't bother to participate. Your kind isn't wanted here.) Baby boards are a wonderful outlet for the stay-at-home mom to feel connected now that dad looks through her, while allowing the working mom to be even less effective on the job. Subject postings include conversational gems such as: *My nipples are bleeding—again!* and *Weird discharge! Pics included.* (Conscientious posters will often include the disclaimer TMI, warning of "too much information" but more accurately interpreted as "too much isolation.")

Finding Your Cyber Soul Sisters

First, it's important to determine which online board is the right group for you. If the page is dotted by pastel bears and cooing infants, you're going to be dealing with the touchy-feely types, generous with homespun advice and emoticons. If there's a banner featuring a stylish and coifed character dressed in heels and toting a handbag, you're dealing with women who *used* to look like that, and who are now more generous with caffeinated critiques and blame.

Still not sure which group suits your sensibilities? Here are some yes-or-no questions to help determine your best online mom match.

- Do you own a Precious Moments figurine? (Camp Cuddly)
- Do you read your horoscope with some shame? (Camp Critical)
- Do you send e-cards? (Camp Cuddly)
- Do you delete e-cards? (Camp Critical)
- Does a relative cut your hair? (Camp Cuddly)
- Is "analysis" part of your household budget? (Camp Critical)
- Do you own a Bible cozy? Any cozy? (Camp Cuddly)

The Dead-Tired Society

Although online baby boards are a convenient way to connect with moms during those overwhelming first weeks, nothing is as bonding as face-to-face time. Welcome to the mommy mixer—think book club, where half of the guests can't control their bowels. Mommy mixers are not only a wonderful excuse to get out of doors, but also a great gathering of women who probably look a little worse than you. You'll recognize them by their stroller clusters, monopolizing most of the aisle space of an already-crowded coffee house or perhaps overtaking one half of a California Pizza Kitchen. The inconsolable crying and rocking are also dead giveaways. And then there are all the babies.

Mommy mixers last usually a total of three weeks, just enough time to realize you have nothing in common with these women other than you all let your guard down around the same time last year. Yes, you all have infants, but after much discussion of Diaper Genies, you'll wish for a *real* genie to help you disappear into a bottle of a different sort. Pretty soon, the group will disband and waiters will happily resume receiving 15 percent gratuities—without having to sweep up a single Cheerio.

Other mommy cults include those women who actually have the gumption to try to get out there and get fit. This group is decidedly more optimistic, naïve in their thinking that baby and yoga have any rightful place together. (An hour of attempted sun salutes while baby wails usually takes care of this notion.) Some opt for "Strollersizing," which is great if baby will remain unconscious long enough for you to break a sweat. (Same rule applies to your sex life.) And if baby does sleep, it only serves to remind you of that missed precious opportunity for you to be unconscious as well. But who has time for a nap? You've got a stroller convoy to lead!

MOMMY ON-SIGHT

A handy field guide for identifying and classifying moms in their natural habitats (malls, grocery stores, Curves, Jenny Craig centers, etc.)

"I Lactate, Therefore I Am": Mammary Mama

Far from discreet, this mom wants—no, *needs*—you to see her boob on display. *Look what a good mother I am*, her protruding spigots proclaim to the chagrin of fellow shoppers and delight of teenage boys. Yes, it's been determined that breast is best if you do it for at least six months. (Otherwise, you're just a poser.) But there are ways to feed your child that don't involve putting those brown Frisbees in the face of others. (Poncho? Giant umbrella?) Clearly, a mom should be able to meet her baby's nutritional needs with flexibility and freedom, but let's not forget one essential fact here: *your tit is out.*

"You Mean You Don't Make Your Own Compost??": Green Mama

This is the mom who loves to borrow trouble—but only organically grown trouble. When she's not toting her naturally woven grocery tote, making you feel like an earth-killing jerk, she's tapping the nearest tree for sap-based diaper balm. She's the one who's up bright and early at the Farmer's Market (the one you thought was an urban legend), and purees her own baby food. She'll usually have baby fastened to her while reeking of herbs and the residual aroma of the natural deodorant that fails her miserably. Most ambitious of all, she uses cloth diapers (see diaper debate on page 94), which speak to both her environmental commitment and olfactory fortitude. Play dates will generally involve planting something, whittling, or, God forbid, volunteering. At holiday time, she's the mom who stuffs fruit in her children's stockings while they pray in vain that this year the banana-shaped protrusion is a boomerang. (Later, her kids will be the ones who come over and ravage your pantry like starving bears.) She is free of both preservatives and joy. If you don't own a hybrid or at least a pair of gardening clogs, don't bother wasting her time. Your Tyrannosaurus-like carbon footprint will far overshadow any possibility of friendship.

"Baby, You Want Another Sip of Coke?": White-Trash Mama

In most cases, this mom had her twenties yanked out from under her by motherhood, but she isn't about to let "some baby" slow her down. She's easily identified by the terrycloth jog suit circa six seasons ago which artfully recedes to reveal her obligatory lower back tattoo. (Roses or cartoon characters figure most prominently. Notable mention: barbed-wire etching around the ankle.) Ensemble is generally accessorized with gas station sunglasses and gigantic cold coffee drink. You'll recognize her child by the pierced hoops that have been dangling from her infant ears since moments after her umbilical was cut. Ask to see a recent baby photo and you'll be confronted with a mascara-coated moppet hopelessly lost in a sea of marabou. She is the answer to the question: who watches the show *Reba?* White-Trash Mama's stroller is as collapsible as her life. Hers is an acid-washed existence. Stay far away and avoid getting burned.

Deciphering the Diaper Bag

Looking for mommy friends? The bag a mom totes says just as much about her as her child's good looks or lack thereof. Here's the lowdown on mommy's baggage.

DESIGNER DIAPER BAG AND/OR LARGE DESIGNER PURSE: Unless she and her child look strikingly alike, chances are you're about to make friends with someone's nanny (who's in charge of the well-being of the bag, as well as baby). Observing her dead stare in the distance as her tiny charge chokes on a coin, she'll only confirm your worst fears about your own sitter. Move on.

GIVEAWAY TOTE:

She got it in the lost-and-found; same place where her baby often turns up. This is a multiple-child mom who's so over it, she'd be just as happy leaving baby on the back of the very bookmobile that sponsored this fashion choice. Note the unraveling edges that speak to the theme of her tattered life. Be a-frayed.

CARTOON-THEMED CARRYALL:

If you want to discuss the difficulties of being a working mom or fitting baby around your Pilates schedule, this isn't a good match. If you want to talk about baby, baby, baby and more about the baby, then start an exchange (not excluding coupon exchange) with this Mombot.

DEALING WITH THE CHILDLESS
Losing Non-Mom Friends

"At first, I felt overwhelmed by visitors. But now that I'm a mom, my friends have virtually dropped off the planet. Will I ever get my social life back, not to mention a normal purse?"

It's natural to feel excluded from normal society when "normal" for you now means wearing vomit as an accessory. This can be especially unnerving if many of your friends don't have children yet. Your new standing as "mom" can make you seems as exotic as some form of West Nile or herpes they pray they never catch. Although your baby will require almost all of your full attention, it's important to remember the person you were before—the person who didn't handle excrement while simultaneously eating lunch. Here are some ways of keeping your street cred with the people you knew back when you were cool.

- Tell brunch pals to think of your child as a shopping bag
- Blame mom brain on being drunk
- Refer to baby as "my bitch"
- Borrow sex-life anecdotes from your sitter's MySpace page

Other Rules of Thumb for Relating to the Barren

- Ban all speak of nipples
- No email photo sharing that involves "signing up" or entering a pass code (not even grandparents care that much)
- No anecdotes involving your child's bodily functions
- Don't suggest lunch at the fast-food playground
- The word "episiotomy" can kill any cocktail gathering

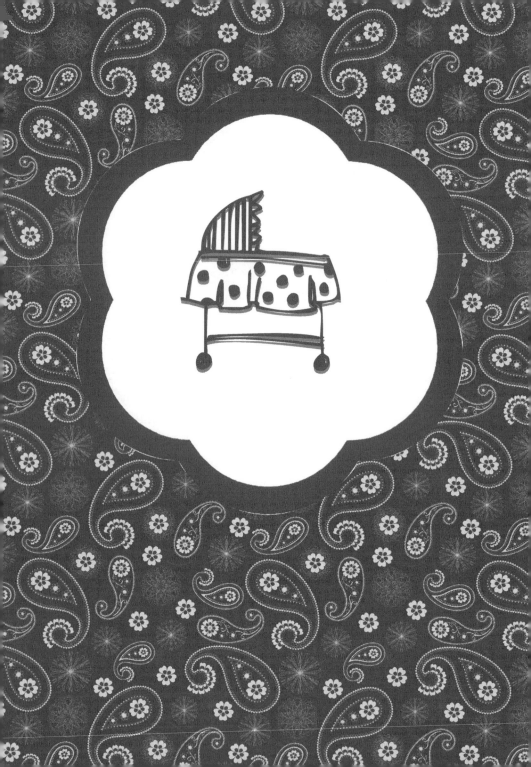

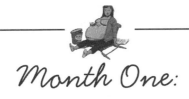

CHAPTER 12

Month One:
"No, I'm Not Pregnant
Anymore—Really."

In the early months, parents tend to live by baby's milestones. It's often the best way to see if your infant is on track and how much you can lord over other babies born around the same time. In the following chapters, the general milestone check will be organized into what a baby better be able to do/most likely will be able to do and may even able to do so you can learn the wide range of normal. Also included throughout the chapters are things baby *cannot* do, so you won't waste time trying to teach your stubby-legged companion how to drive stick.

HOW FAR YOUR BABY LAGS BEHIND OTHERS
By One Month, Baby...
...BETTER BE ABLE TO:

Concentrate on people, but only appropriately attractive ones.

...MOST LIKELY WILL BE ABLE TO:
React to a noise like an oven timer—with expressions that convey "turn off that goddamn oven timer."

...MAY EVEN:
Raise head in order to breathe and save you messy allegations.

...WON'T BE ABLE TO:
Make your DUI go away.

FORTY-EIGHT HOURS AND EVERYONE IS STILL ALIVE!

A couple of days after you bring baby home, he'll be scheduled for a follow-up exam. This is a time when your doctor can check that baby is thriving and that you didn't run out on the bill. The second week check-up is to ensure you're meeting baby's needs and didn't leave him on top of the car at the last appointment. In fact, just showing up with the baby is half of the exam.

WHAT YOU MAY BE FREAKED OUT ABOUT
Where's The Handle on This Thing?

"I'm worried I'll accidentally hurt my newborn. You should see the condition of my designer handbag—and that cost me thousands."

With a wobbly head and floppy limbs, your baby may appear breakable—if not extremely lazy—but really, baby is one tough customer. Essentially, apply the same care to baby's head as you would your favorite sunglasses—minus enveloping in a case, of course.

In-Vogue Infant?

"My baby appears to be losing weight, but the doctor's scale shows a steady increase. I'm sure my baby looks thinner. Is it just wishful thinking?"
Congratulations for getting a baby with a little self-discipline. While other mothers have to tote little tubs of lard, you can relax in sheer smugness—your baby would rather gag himself on his rattle (another effective slimming technique) than be caught dead with carb-face. So how does he do it? Notice how baby attempts to push up when put on his chest. How else do you think he rocks his triceps? Reaching for mobile? Total core blast. This doesn't even include his liquid diet. Rightfully, you should pity those mothers with babies whose arms and legs look like tied-off balloons. Go ahead and ask them for their short-sleeved onesies. They won't be needing them.

Sorry, Recreational Use Only

"I've been breast-feeding my daughter for a month, but now I'm ready to call it off and use a bottle. Of course, I plan to lie to all my friends about it, but I still can't shake feeling guilty!"
You're right to feel guilty. No telling what you've done to the appearance of your breasts. Luckily, you became aware in enough time to stop your rack drop mid-plunge. Just use a little duct tape for day and low lighting and your spouse's fertile imagination by night. (Different shape and density will be like touching a whole new woman. At least that's how his mental script usually plays out.) If all goes well, you may still be able to wear a bikini with pride.

Or just get great big fake ones. Then you'll finally be happy. We promise.

Li'l Lestat

"My baby spends daylight hours snoozing, but perks up when the sun goes down. And I hate late-night television. How do I get her on a normal schedule?"

It's like living with your meth-addicted roommate all over again, isn't it?* You can be assured that baby will work out her internal clock soon enough. Until that time, try keeping her from napping for more than a couple of hours in a stretch. Of course, waking a sleeping baby is sometimes easier said than done. Below are some techniques to help keep your drowsy little angel from sleepyville.

- Marinate teether in habanera sauce.
- Wild, barking dogs. Every hour on the hour.
- Install TMX surround-sound in bassinet.
- Use megaphone as cozy swaddler. Whisper "wake up" from the mouth end.

Baby, You're a Star

"Is it possible my baby is gifted? If so, when will he begin to show signs? He's somewhat unattractive, so we've got fingers crossed."

By the mere fact you asked, the answer is no. Don't you know that most gifted children are born of plain folk who never think to question the aptitude of their children? (Or the authority of the man in the household.) But if you must find out if your child will possibly cure the future celebrity-endorsed disease or invent the next bad-ass computer game, here are some cues to look for as he develops.

---

*Except for the stealing-your-money-and-burning-alive-in-a-meth-lab part.

AS EARLY AS SIX MONTHS:
- Baby is only soothed by lulling sounds of NPR
- Black-and-white shapes—like *The Wall Street Journal*—captivate him
- Baby cries when the NASDAQ plunges

AS EARLY AS A YEAR:
- Baby uses blocks to spell out desires like "AVOID A STATE SCHOOL"
- Baby answers the phone using clear enunciation (but forgets to take a message)
- Baby gets correct answers on *Jeopardy* but fails to put in form of a question

BY PRESCHOOL:
- Baby finds loophole for $5000 tax savings
- Baby balances economy while watching *Go, Diego, Go*
- Baby develops quantum physics theory that relegates Stephen Hawking to campy television cameos

Linus-Itis

"Our one-month-old baby is starting to show signs of dependency on a particular blanket. He has trouble sleeping without it. We're considering taking it away so he won't live with us when he's thirty."

You're right to intervene now. One month old is far too old to be relying on childish accoutrement like blankets, bears, and pacifiers. He'll be a total joke by three months and rightfully shunned if the adults and children around him have any standards. What's next?

Calling his mother "ma-ma?" *Shudder.* Given your attentiveness to the matter, baby has nothing to be insecure about. He can be fully confident his parents will be alongside him every step of the way—critiquing his walking attempts, scaring away potential friends, and writing his college term papers. Clearly, you only want what's best for your son. At least that is what you can tell him as you're trying to coax him to surrender the gun and come down from the top of the tower.

camera Shy?

"When I try to take a picture, baby instantly shuts her eyes. Help! Her career as a child model is at stake!"

Blinking at a bright light doesn't exactly make baby a vampire. Chances are you've paparazzied the kid's pupils into permanent constriction. Lay off, Herb Ritts, and give baby a moment. You're not exactly going to be selling these to the *National Enquirer* (and your friends are *so* over your online photo barrage). Step away from the Snapfish, and take in your baby outside of the lens. Chances are she'll gaze right back at the blurry figure her seared retinas process as you. Now that's a Kodak moment.

Bless You, Messing with You

"Why does my baby constantly sneeze? Really, it's so annoying. Could it be allergies already?"

Faker. Your baby is exhibiting the earliest signs of hypochondria. Don't fall for it. Those sneezes are merely cries for attention (also listen for the faux sneeze where she's actually calling you an *"ass-HOLE"*). Other faker baby signatures: pretending to have poor coordination and smiling and laughing at nothing particularly witty or droll. From this point on, when baby sneezes, greet her with a stern, "You know what you did." Expect your child to persist by acting confused well into adulthood. Never give in to the mind games. *Never.* Who's the *"ass-HOLE"* now?

KEEPING BABY IN ONE PIECE: BEYOND BABY-PROOFING

Although most babies stay healthy and happy, all it takes is an unattended Roomba or a neighbor's pet python and you've got a 911 call on your hands. To help your child stay out of harm's way, follow all of these rules all of the time.

- Always strap baby in. Have your local fire station check the car seat installation (Surprise! Many firefighters aren't the sexy gay men you see posing in calendars.) And never let an infant drive. The neck is too weak to support their head, and they can't quite discern colors yet. No matter what the circumstance, a cop is never going to buy that "I can only see shades of black and white, Officer" excuse.

- Avoid placing baby seats where they could topple. It's the adult equivalent of placing your own chair precariously on a table—while drunk. Like last Tuesday.

- No rough and sudden jostling of baby, no matter how much loose change you think you'll find.

- No matter how fast you can pee, don't leave baby by himself. It only takes seconds for a baby to make an adult selection on your cable box or purchase a Bowflex.

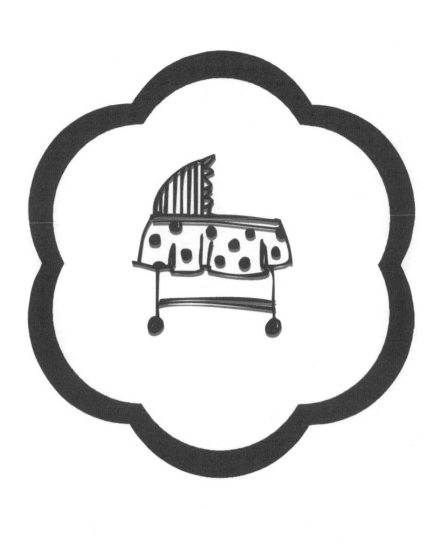

CHAPTER 13

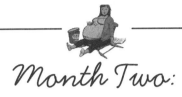

Month Two:
Hygiene, Interrupted

If baby is still alive, congratulations. You've done a hell of a job. Of course, your marriage is likely D.O.A., but don't worry. No one is going anywhere for a while. By now, baby's cervix-squashed ears have unfolded, hinting at the identity of the real father. You're probably feeling like a baby pro, able to simultaneously talk on the phone and rescue your little one only minutes after she is trapped under a smothering blanket. Your nights are probably sleepless due to feedings, a welcome exchange from the wakeful evenings staring at the window wondering if he's with that bitch. Of course, you haven't crossed the finish line yet, sleepyhead. You've got years of PTA meetings, theme restaurants, joyless sex, and disastrous affairs ahead of you. That will help keep you awake.

HOW FAR YOUR BABY LAGS BEHIND OTHERS
As before mentioned, all babies reach a new stage whenever the hell they want to.

But if baby is behind on more than one of these, he probably has a wilderness boot camp in his future. (For a head start, practice saying, "It's because I love you! It's because I love you!")

By Two Months, Baby...

...BETTER BE ABLE TO:
Mirror a smile—even fake ones.

...MOST LIKELY WILL BE ABLE TO:
Mumble (cooing or humming catchy tunes).

...MAY EVEN:
Notice the little things, such as loose Vicodin floating in your couch cushions.
Grab at devices such as the phone.

...WON'T BE ABLE TO:
Get your take-out order right.

WELL-BABY CHECK: LET THE SCORE-KEEPING COMMENCE

These are called well-baby checks because the doctor usually begins each exam with, "Well, baby. Ready to jump back inside?"* The organization of the exam and procedures performed will vary depending on whether or not you've finally wised up about all that holistic crap. Here's what to expect at a regular baby exam.

---

*Get in line behind dad.

- Questions about baby's assimilation and if doctor can finally tell his black-market connection with some certainty, "the bluebird has flown"
- Record of weight gain and head circumference to note changes in growth and baby's level of arrogance
- React and Respond: a prick test (doctor will poke baby's foot to see if he reacts like a total jerk)

Practice for Talk Therapy Later

When you hear those adorable babbling consonants ("ba-ba"; "ga-ga"; "na-na") it's no longer your partner coming down from a bad trip. It's the beginning of language, baby's first attempt to save himself from inept care. (Example: ga-ga-ga: phonetic beginning of *"ga-ga...got* to get out of here"; *"ba-ba...ba*-d idea being born; "na-na...911.")

WHAT YOU MAY BE FREAKED OUT ABOUT
English as a Second Language

Tired of yelling *"What?" "What?"* to your babbling, incoherent infant? At times, you're not sure who's more intelligible—your baby or your barely English-proficient housekeeper who keeps referring to the kitchen as "the chicken." Sure, you've tried getting on his level by watching the same shows and matching him bottle for bottle, but still the communication divide exists. That's because most of what baby is telling you is nonverbal. The key is observation: keen, unflinching, staring-closely-while-they-sleep, going through their pockets—okay, that's someone else. Anyway, watch baby with some regularity, and you'll get the picture.

Keep Talking. And Talking.

BE A NARRATOR

Dictate your daily routine: "Now I'm going to the medicine cabinet to take a Claritin. No, Mommy doesn't have allergies. It's the only nonprescription that will jack me up enough to crawl through this purgatory called a day. See, if it's not prescribed then it's not a problem." Describe washing dishes, ironing the clothes, vacuuming, cooking dinner, and how in one fell swoop, you managed to go back in time fifty years. Baby won't be able to understand a word of it, but your desperate tone will serve as a subconscious cautionary tale about the pitfalls of extended maternity leave.

ASK BABY

It's never too early to start Q& A. "Do you think Daddy finds our next-door neighbor more attractive than me?"; "Once I shed about fifteen pounds, do you think teenage boys would consider me hot?" Go as far as to even answer yourself on behalf of baby. "Should I follow his car tonight or should we stay in and read a story? Follow the car? Great idea!"

THERE'S NO "I" IN "BABY"

Babies will be quicker to identify people if you refer to them with words like "Mommy," "Daddy," or "Neighborhood Tramp."

BABY CAN'T TELL TIME

Baby lives in the moment. Like the night that bartender slipped you a roofie, baby has no concept of the past or future.

MAKE TIME FOR STORY TIME

Feel free to indulge in favorite books from your own childhood with their outdated racist and sexist overtones. ("Oh, Brer Rabbit, how you remind me of the good ol' days of the South;" "Cinderella doesn't need a degree—she has a prince!") Or if you crave adult-level entertainment, you can indulge in your regular reading fare. "Marcia had tamed her share of cowboys, but the front expanse between his well-worn chaps revealed a denim saddle horn that begged to be gripped…"

UNEXPECTED TIPS FOR CREATING A COCOON BABY WILL NEVER WANT TO LEAVE
How to Love Your Baby and Get Baby to Love You Back...

OFFER UNCONDITIONAL AFFECTION

Nothing says love like staying around for good behavior as well as when there's hitting and biting. This will be very important for your child to remember for her relationships later. Specifically, offer the same patient love you did to your alcoholic boyfriend all those years. That wasn't wasted, right?

FIND COMMON GROUND WITH BABY

Let baby know you have tons in common outside of that previous umbilical cord connection. ("You like juice? I like juice!"; "You need air?" "So do I!") Try laughing when baby laughs ("Giraffes?

Hysterical! Their necks are absurdly long!") and taking up baby's hobbies and interests. ("Ahh! That jack-in-the-box always scares the bejeezus out of me, too!"; "Bears really are one big hairy hug....")

PLAY HARD TO GET

It's important to create an air of mystery with baby and not be too available. (Another lesson learned so many restraining orders ago.) Have baby seek *you* out and decide which cries you want to respond to (hunger) and which cries you choose to ignore (crouching housecat).

BE BABY'S CHEERLEADER

When your baby achieves something (grasps a rattle, lifts himself up) respond with huge gesticulations and praise. It's important to instill in baby that everything he does is wonderful. The future women he leaves in his wake will have you to thank for it, not including all the impossible friends and employers who "just don't get him."

TIMING IS EVERYTHING

Keep in mind, babies have a short attention span, so always bring your best material. This is no time to phone it in. Sixteen hours of sleep a day doesn't leave baby much time to endure lackluster performances. If you want to establish a real connection, some times are better than others. For example, when *Maisy* is on, you're dead to baby. Wait until baby is hungry and wear her bottle around your neck. Then you'll have her complete attention. Notice the high-pitch wailing and desperate reach. See, baby is crazy about you!

THE UNEXPECTED FIELD GUIDE FOR MAKING BABY'S TINY BRAIN BIGGER

To some, depending on the immaturity of their spouse, participation in play can come very naturally. Other parents struggle with baby activities ("I don't even like blocks. Why are we stacking them? Yeah, they fell over. What's so hilarious?") Here are some areas of exploration for you and your pint-sized play partner.

A Tasting

Baby's taste buds are doing just that—budding—so likely they want to tongue-explore (not the same way you did that summer practicing kissing at the all-girls camp). Try not to discourage baby unless it's something poisionous or a choking hazard. As much as it may gross you out, this is a way of learning about the world, just like you calmly tried to explain to the camp counselor while having to pack your things.

The Sniffer

You may not realize it, but baby's nose is getting a workout every day. All kinds of new aromas are invading his air space: Mommy's lotion, Daddy's failures. Unless baby is being suffocated by those vanilla volcanoes you call candles, then let him continue to follow his nose.

Peepers

Far from being blind at birth, we now know babies can not only see, but judge. Within hours, baby can determine you from a chair, a terrifically useful tool especially if they're left to wander in a furniture store. From the very beginning, it's important to maximize baby's visual senses through his surroundings. Try painting one side of the nursery in bold vivid colors, or hire a nanny who is extremely good looking. Other items can provide additional stimulus: disco balls, flashing lights, and again, dynamic prints and colors. In other words, just imagine baby is gay. Not only will your infant get the visual stimulation he needs, you'll benefit from his campy humor and impeccable sense of style. Now on cue, exchange play swats: *"Oh you!"*

OTHER EXCITING SIGHTS:

- Mirrors: Babies love gazing at their own image. When baby learns it's her in the mirror, you can show her that tiny irregular mole on her cheek while assuring her that "makeup will do a fine job of hiding it." Keep pointing this out well into her teen years.
- Family albums: Walk baby down the memory lane that led you straight to intensive therapy. A family photo album is the perfect opportunity to show her who she got her sweet dimples from, as well as the genetic predisposition for cocktails before 11 a.m. (thanks, Grandma!)
- Household objects: Sounds crazy, but baby likes to stare at things around the house that you wouldn't think twice about. So don't feel odd about "time with toaster" or "getting to know Mr. Coffee." They are as exciting as your remaining friends who are falling away with each passing day. Bonus? If estranged from loved ones, feel free to adopt Aunt Jemima or Uncle Ben as nurturing family

figures. (Mrs. Butterworth can serve as adorable kooky neighbor.) You've got a pantry full of love and you didn't even know it.

- The people and things outside his door: Taking baby out in a stroller or face-forward in a carrier can give him early and welcome exposure to his place on this planet. Feel free to narrate as you go along the sidewalk: "See that man urinating against the building? We do that in our diapers. Yes we do!"; "There's a woman headed to work. Daddy says Mommy should go back to work, but we have a surprise for him, don't we?"

Can You Hear Me Now?

Hearing is how baby learns about language and music, and your best friend's affair with her yoga instructor.

USING YOUR VOICE:

It's the most important auditory influence in your baby's life, so talk and talk some more to baby. It can be about anything: the people around you, what is going on in your life, even made-up stories. So essentially, it's a lot like brunch. For even more auditory exposure, imitate other familiar sounds, like the bark of the dog you abandoned in the backyard, or your cat's meow. ("Do we still have a cat?")

CHILDREN'S MUSIC:

Get ready to revisit your favorite bands from the '80s and '90s who had to make that mortgage payment once the royalty checks ran out. As a result, today's kiddie music actually has a pleasant tone that overrides the desperate one emanating from these now-career-defunct crooners. Sure, Frankie Goes to Hollywood, but what happens when *"Frankie Goes Potty?"* Honestly, there's nothing like listening to the songs you used to get high to, remastered for your children's enjoyment. (Example: "The Roof Is on Fire" becomes "The Roosters Aren't Tired!" Genius.) Can't get enough soulful ballads about brushing your teeth and peanut butter and jelly? *"Relax!"* Operators are standing by…

SING-SONG PLAYTHINGS:
Singing snakes or monkeys that make music when you pull their tail will not only intrigue your child but will also leave him dangerously misinformed about the animal world. (If your little one suffers from fever and chills after a trip to the zoo, check for symmetric puncture wounds.) The most important rule of thumb for musical makers is to make sure they're not too startling or loud for sensitive ears. That means no "Ozzy-in-a-box" or " Cuddle Me KISS bears."

The Tactile Experience

Touch is baby's most important tool to connect with others. How often they are touched is how baby knows Mommy, her scruffy-faced Daddy, and, years later, when it's time to seek marriage counseling. When you hold and cuddle your baby, you're letting him know one thing for sure: *Enjoy it now, buddy. No one will ever be as good to you as I am.*

Here are some touch experiences that will stay with your child for a lifetime.

RUB-A-DUB, NOT IN TUB:
Studies show that babies who regularly receive full-body massages tend to thrive more often than babies who opt for quick chair massage. Because your baby is so delicate, it's best to avoid anything more intensive than the gentle hand of Mommy or Daddy. Remember, that hot-stone massage you enjoy is like a smoldering boulder-crushing for baby. And no deep tissue. It feels good at the time but always makes baby so damn sore the next day.

FEELING GOOD AROUND THE HOUSE:
Try exposing baby to different textures and explaining each (cashmere: good; polyester blends: bad.) Place baby on his tummy and let him experience each surface directly—grandma's fur coat, the cool marble countertop, the scratchy tiles of your house roof, the soft gurney of the children's E.R....

TOUCHY-FEELY TOYS:
Now playtime can be a tactile adventure. Corduroy bears or wooden cars will alert and interest baby; a prickly cactus or bag of nails will alert and interest authorities.

NURTURING IN THE NURSERY
Socialization

Your baby learns about socialization by watching you interact with others. But that doesn't mean baby is going to be throwing dinner parties and calling your sister a bitch after two drinks. Baby will first start by interacting with toys. Think your social clique has issues? Clearly, you have yet to navigate the complex psychological dynamics of the Bratz hierarchy.

Learning How to control that Thing that Keeps Hitting My Face

Right now baby wants you to think his hand movements are innocent flailings ("Did he just shoot me the finger? Nah, it couldn't be...") but within a few months, baby won't be able to play dumb. You can help end the charade by allowing plenty of opportunities to demonstrate the dexterity of his little hands—from picking up blocks to getting that spot on your back you never can seem to reach. And help baby get a handle by not restricting his movements. Confinement can inhibit baby. (Ironic, since such confinements can uninhibit Mommy.)

Learning to Not Fall on My ASS

Babies who get increased muscular strength early tend to have lots of opportunities for self-motivated physical activity ("Want your bottle, kid? It's *way* over there...") You can encourage these developments by letting baby lie tummy-down on your shins. Motivate him to move by not shaving for a day or two before. That, or paint terrifying faces on each of your knees.

Baby's Smarts

Honing of all of the above senses will ultimately aid in cognitive development. Otherwise, start with basic health concerns. To maximize intellectual growth, you'll want to eliminate lead or the CBS television line-up from your child's consumption.

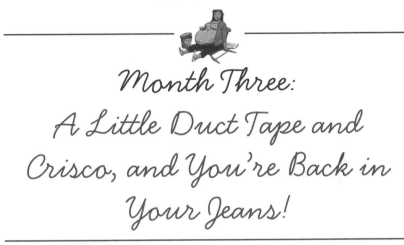

CHAPTER 14

Month Three: A Little Duct Tape and Crisco, and You're Back in Your Jeans!

This month, baby explores a world outside of eating and crying. You will reach this stage much later in the postpartum journey. His hand has become the most wondrous play toy he could have ever imagined. Likewise for his long-ignored father.

HOW FAR YOUR BABY LAGS BEHIND OTHERS
By Three Months, Baby...

...BETTER BE ABLE TO:
Do a spot-on impression of a bag of flour.

...MOST LIKELY WILL BE ABLE TO:
Giggle (but, like Grandpa, at nothing in particular).

...MAY EVEN:
Mock others.

Turn over (and, in the case of approaching grandmother, play dead).

...WON'T BE ABLE TO:
Program your universal remote.

WELL-BABY CHECK: "WELL, YOU'RE STILL A BABY..."

Mountains of relief—at least on the part of the doctor's office. You and your Internet printouts aren't scheduled for a checkup this month.

WHAT YOU MAY BE FREAKED OUT ABOUT
Shake-n-Babe

"My baby can't grab anything! His movements are all jerky. Clearly, he got it from my husband's side, but what should I do?"

Three months and you've already labeled your baby a "jerk"? Congratulations on winning Mother of the Year. Far from being a little weirdo-in-training, baby probably just feels nervous around your ever-critical eye. All babies at this age are uncoordinated, so don't get too upset when baby gets clobbered during a round of golf or table tennis. (And for chrissake, don't bet on him!) Before you know it he'll be able to reach for his bear, hold his bottle, or cut your brake line.

child's Play?

"My husband likes to toss our baby around, but I worry that it will cause permanent damage. He says I'm overreacting, between mouthfuls of kids' cereal. Am I?"

You're right to be concerned. Baby could easily land on Daddy's head or, worse, throw up on him in mid-toss. There are all sorts of unseen adult hazards that can result at the hands of these tiny ruffians, so it's best to exercise caution.

Speaking in Tongues

"My wife's family only speaks Spanish—and she encourages it with our baby. Beyond the little I've picked up from Dora, I only speak English. Won't it cause language confusion?"

There will be no more confusion than already exists in your household. You can argue in any language and baby will get the message loud and clear: she has a lot of work to do if this thing is going to last. What will be more important is your infant's fluency in navigating that land mine of a marriage. She can start by:

FAKING A MAJOR LEARNING DELAY:
Parents will have to bond together to conquer "baby's inability to discern humans from animals." (Warning: unless, of course, it backfires and they point blame.)

COMMITTING A CRIME:
Mom and Dad will need to align baby's alibi and, thus, align hearts.

SECURING A LUCRATIVE MODELING CONTRACT:
They'll be forced to band together if they want to ride baby's gravy train.

GETTING CPS INVOLVED:

Hurling allegations at the couple will get parents on the defensive and, with some luck, on each other.

Unexpected Challenges:
The Constantly Cranky Baby

For some parents, their baby seems born with a chip on its shoulder (and not the tasty, crunchy kind). While you dreamed of a cooperative cooer, you instead got eight pounds of attitude that can't control its bowels. Difficult babies come in all shapes and forms and learning which kind of contender you've got on your hands is the first step to containing them. Here are the types of infant instigators and how you can put baby in a corner.

PROZAC BABY

"Waa-waa" might as well be "waaa-waaan." Your little Debbie Downer always seems to look on the bleak side of things. While other babies delight in their floor gyms or musical mobiles, your tiny pessimist is staring off into the distance, thinking about the hole in the ozone, then crying for no apparent reason. At least, that's how it appears. Try telling her that Al Gore has the environment covered. Expect more crying, this time about the fact that he refuses to run.

DRUG-ADDICT BABY

Or so his behavior would indicate. While most babies are peacefully asleep, your baby is wide awake, wanting to go out for pancakes at 3 a.m. In the end, he'll settle for the breast or the bottle—also not unlike a drug addict. Sort of like parenting an even more pint-sized Andy Dick (minus the going-for-breasts part). The trick is letting baby know he isn't in charge by reorienting him to the household power structure. That might take a few hard lessons. Try placing baby in front of a bowl of delicious Chinese food with—chopsticks! Can't exactly enjoy that Asian goodness without effective hand-eye coordination, can you? And checking email isn't so easy with those stubby little fingers. Pretty soon, baby will understand you can't really rule the world from your parent's perch. Just ask George W. Bush.

LOUD BABY

Your baby can be heard a mile away. Not to mention the carbondated members of your building's co-op board are plotting to have him ousted at the next meeting. A polite way to put it would be "high-spirited" but face it—he's just freakin' loud. One way to rein in your little screamer is challenge him decibel for decibel. Can his little lung capacity compete with the hard licks of The J. Geils Band? You and 15A are about to find out.

Gaa-Gaa, Can't Go There

"Most of my friends talk up a storm to their infants, but I feel ridiculous. Frankly, we don't have a thing in common. He brings nothing to the table but a giant mess. Is our divide going to hurt his growth?"

There's nothing wrong with wanting baby to come to your level. It does seem unfair that you're suddenly forced to speak in the same affectionate tone to this stranger as you would to your dog that you've known for years. One way to get past feeling like a blubbering idiot is to try secondhand dialogue. Try saying things *about* your baby to your spouse, like:

- "Hey. He's still here."
- "Being that bald must be hell in the sun."
- "Do you suppose he gets that shapeless ass from my side of the family?"

My Baby's Bigger Than Yours

"When I pick up my son at daycare, I always run into other parents, who love to compare babies. I notice it's more prevalent among the moms who haven't gotten their bodies back. How can I avoid the "my baby is better " debate and still keep mom friends?"

Afraid of a little friendly competition? Oh, then your baby must be lagging *way* behind. But that's okay. Those babies moving at a faster clip will be happy to tutor your "little fighter." Notice how the moms are drawn to you and your infant. Nothing speaks more to developmental progress than trouncing the next-weaker child. There are ways to put your progeny ahead of the pack, though. You just have to know how to play dirty. Here are some pointers to shut those tit-for-tat moms down for good:

- Overtly massage baby's wrists. When asked, say she's been getting carpal tunnel from writing her latest novel.
- When asked for a play date, pull out your calendar and muse, "Well, we have violin on Tuesdays, Fun with Foreign Policy on Wednesdays…"
- Instead of teether, have baby gnaw on Emmy award.

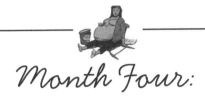

CHAPTER 15

Month Four:
Now That Baby Can Smile at People, You No Longer Exist

Finally, baby has a little personality. Rather than a flesh-and-blood blob sucking you dry of your vital essence, he's occasionally flashing a grin—followed by sucking you dry of your vital essence.

HOW FAR YOUR BABY LAGS BEHIND OTHERS
By Four Months, Baby...

...BETTER BE ABLE TO:

Turn away from your unsightly choice of lounge wear.

Focus on something specific—especially if it's his bottle, and he's starving.

...MOST LIKELY WILL BE ABLE TO:

Survey surroundings and then collapse in disappointment.

...MAY EVEN:

Look up when he hears someone talking, particularly someone who says, "I'm your real mother."

Protest if you take something away and subsequently plan scathing memoir about you.

...WON'T BE ABLE TO:

Bridge the gap between you and your estranged parents.

WELL-BABY CHECK: "HERE, YOU HOLD HER DURING THE SHOT SO SHE'LL HATE YOU INSTEAD."

It's been a whole two months since your doctor has given you that one-on-one time you so desperately crave, and boy, is she in for it. Along with weight, length, and head measurements, immunizations are also on the schedule. This in mind, it's best to get your many questions out of the way first, before baby is riddled with holes and in no mood for your needy crap.

WHAT YOU MAY BE FREAKED OUT ABOUT
Breast Intentions

"My baby was a breast-feeding champ, but all of a sudden he's lost interest. Is my milk bad? My husband says it tastes fine."

Not likely. Baby is getting older and it probably dawned on him: *Dear God. What am I doing??* This is why most people can't remember anything before the age of two. It's nature's way of erasing this embarrassing blunder between parent and child. Much like alcohol works for adults. You have to give your child due credit. Unlike you, baby knows what boobs are for—careers in television and to land someone rich enough to allow you to be a stay-at-home whatever.

It's All Relative

"My mother and mother-in-law are constantly debating my baby's routine. One tells me I need to set it in stone, the other says be flexible. Which of these know-it-all bitches is right?"

As usual, neither. Every baby is different, so it varies. Some babies will be early birds and some will want to sleep off the hangover that is infanthood. That said, here is a schedule your little one might impose if he had any say in the matter:

6 a.m.: Wake just long enough for Mommy to ingest at least two cups of coffee so it's impossible for her to go back to sleep. Suck down a bottle or chew Mommy's nipples into knobs of hamburger meat. Change me, dammit.

8 a.m.: One more milk/formula hit and go back to sleep. Dream about sheep, duckies, teddy bears…the stuff that we babies think about all day. Need another change. Trying to call for assistance but this goddamn phone keeps connecting me to farm animals.

10 a.m.: Endure the new and "friendlier" version of Martha Stewart with Mommy. Cover heart in case Martha leaps out of television and rips it from my tiny chest. (When I grow up, I'm going to become a director of television programming and ban any show that panders to a studio audience. On this bear, I swear it.)

11 a.m.: Liquid lunch then nap. Pray that Mommy uses down time for overdue shower.

1 p.m.: Wake for another bottle/boob hit. Play in Exersaucer and watch Mommy make a series of desperate calls to friends at work who have no time to chat.

3 p.m.: Have another bottle and watch Mommy call Daddy at work and tell him all about my day. Call is cut short. After a bye-bye and hang-up, she calls him "a prick." (Note to self: Google "prick" after dinner.)

4 p.m.: Take a loop around the neighborhood in stroller. Meet up with other moms who look a little worse than Mommy—then again, I'm prejudiced. Try to tune out talk about car seats and those pesky last ten pounds while watching them pound thousand-calorie coffee drinks. *Duh*.

6 p.m.: Dinner. Knocked back 8 oz. Going to be soooo fat!

8 p.m.: Think about going to bed. But good television is coming on, and I know Mommy and Daddy want me awake for that. Soon they will return me and my stuffed animals to big white jail. Thinking of pulling an "Escape from Alcatraz" but need to get my hands on a ripe melon that resembles my head. Luckily, at this hairless juncture, the choices are endless. Plan in place. Elmo and the bunnies are on their own.

10 p.m.: Last bottle and straining to stay awake. Some stupid couples-in-crisis show is on, and the characters are whining about how they never sex anymore. Watch Mommy and Daddy grow extremely uncomfortable. I get to sleep in their bed, after all!

1 a.m.: Wake as soon as Mommy's deep REM cycle sets in. Repeat as necessary.

Giving Baby Props

"I was out and about with my baby when I was lectured by an elderly woman who said she wasn't old enough to be sitting upright up in a stroller. As a precautionary measure, I told her to go screw herself, but was she on to something?"

Old people. They can be so annoying. No wonder they are going extinct. And in this situation, your gray-haired friends are in the wrong. A baby who holds his head up can and should be positioned to see the world. Plus, from such a vantage point, they can signal when another meddlesome octogenarian approaches. With a simple, "Look, there's a baby without a hat, and it's 70 degrees out!" or "Hey, another survivor from the *Andrea Doria!*" they'll instantly become distracted, and you can easily make your escape. Or you can install a cowcatcher to your stroller as a preventive measure to ward off those pesky purse-clutchers.

Baby Gap?

"My baby loves to bounce on my lap. It's the only thing that keeps her happy. Can this deform her legs?"

Baby won't become deformed. But there are indicators that baby is already paving a career path. Specifically, does baby also salivate at the sight of money in small denominations? Does she laugh at men's jokes whether they're funny or not? Does she insist on having you refer to her stroller as the Camaro? Congratulations! You've got yourself a little stripper-in-training. Now all baby needs is a great story about why this is temporary (it's not) and a place to lock away all her hopes and dreams. (Camaro trunk?)

THE UNEXPECTED FIELD GUIDE FOR PLAYING WITH BABY
Baby Toys

Walking down a toy aisle, there are a host of irresistible choices, sort of like walking down a liquor aisle. ("Hey kids! It's Captain Morgan! Well, he's sort of like Cap'n Crunch back when he used to get laid.") Although such a selection can bring out the kid in anyone, there are things you must keep in mind before you "Sit 'n Spin" down memory lane.

IS IT SUITABLE FOR BABY'S DEVELOPMENTAL LEVEL?
Baby's got years before she'll master a Nintendo or need the companionship of the Rabbit Pearl (Mommies, you know what we're talking about). It's best to check the box for age appropriateness. You don't want that robotic monkey sitting in your house intellectually intimidating your child, nor do you want a juvenile lawn mower/bubble blower limiting his future to the landscaping arts.

IS IT ENGAGING?
Toys should appeal to all of the senses: visual senses (mirror: yes; magnifying glass in sun: no); hearing (a music box: yes; iPod: no).

COULD IT BE HAZARDOUS?
Toys are responsible for countless injuries each year, so it's important to know whether you're setting baby up for a head start or a headstone. Toys should be well-made and meet industry standards so avoid any "make your own trampoline" kits or rifle/pogo-stick combos.

IS IT OKAY FOR SNUGGLING?

Children love to cuddle animals. But before baby embraces a real bear or oh-so-huggable raccoon, they should practice on stuffed toy animals. Sure, they may not be equipped with tooth and claw, but their make-believe counterparts should be treated with similar caution:

- To avoid choking hazards, eyes and noses should not be made of buttons, gemstones, or aspirin.
- No wire insides, especially barbed or electric.
- No strings. For example, teddy bear can't require love under just any circumstance.
- Check for durability so stuffing won't come out. You don't want baby poking around on the real Fido looking for his foam insides.
- Plush toys should never be placed in baby's crib. They are made for receiving affection; thus, they can suffocate baby in secret agenda to get all the love in the house.

MORE OF WHAT YOU MAY BE FREAKED OUT ABOUT

Latch-Free Kid

"My daughter wails like a banshee when we buckle her in the car. I keep telling her buying a Suburban wasn't my idea."

Have you considered she's reacting to your driving? From her rear-facing vantage, you appear to always be headed straight into the car in front of you. She lays on her fake horn, but to no avail. Screaming, she is just anticipating the overdue impact to which you seem oblivious. Other possible sources of discomfort:

- Forced to stare at the car's fabric interior, she worries why you couldn't afford leather.
- She can't remove that blasted toy latched to the car seat arm.
- She considers "mirror baby" evil arch nemesis.
- She's forced to stare straight into sunlight à la Clockwork Orange because that half-assed suction-cup sun shield keeps falling.

Back Talk

"My baby hates sleeping on his back. But I hear it's the best way to guard against SIDS—and witches."

There can be a host of reasons baby hates being on his back. Often on-the-tummy is downright more comfortable. But perhaps there are other reasons baby can't nod off. Here are a couple of possible reasons to check:

- Baby thinks decorative ceiling fan is machete-armed killing machine.
- Baby is obsessed with precariously attached chandelier dangling above crib in slow, twisting death spiral.
- Baby lives in terror of creepy clown-head finials.

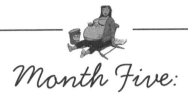

CHAPTER 16

Month Five:
Finally Sent out Those Birth Announcements!

By now, your baby has a look and personality that is all his own. Unfortunately, you've spent the last few months boring everyone with so many updates that they no longer care.

HOW FAR YOUR BABY LAGS BEHIND OTHERS

As always emphasized in these pages, babies reach their own milestones at a different pace. If your baby is a little behind or not quite on the mark, she's in good company—if you define "alone" as in good company.

By Five Months, Baby...

...BETTER BE ABLE TO:

Hold his head up in moments where you don't embarrass him. Smile at you, then make a disgusted face as you turn away.

...MOST LIKELY WILL BE ABLE TO:

Make babbling noises that you can falsely claim as a first word.

...MAY EVEN:

Balance with some assistance—preferably not a skittish pet or feeble elderly family member.

Pretend to reach for a toy and con you into doing it for him.

...WON'T BE ABLE TO:

Organize his uncle's intervention.

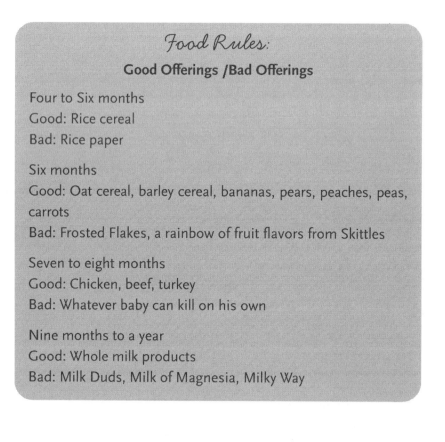

Food Rules:
Good Offerings /Bad Offerings

Four to Six months
Good: Rice cereal
Bad: Rice paper

Six months
Good: Oat cereal, barley cereal, bananas, pears, peaches, peas, carrots
Bad: Frosted Flakes, a rainbow of fruit flavors from Skittles

Seven to eight months
Good: Chicken, beef, turkey
Bad: Whatever baby can kill on his own

Nine months to a year
Good: Whole milk products
Bad: Milk Duds, Milk of Magnesia, Milky Way

WELL-BABY CHECK: THE DOCTOR IS IN...LUCK

Nothing. Your pediatrician finally gets another break from your paranoid ass.

Store up all that craziness for next month.

BABY TAKES A BITE
Big Food, Big Problems

Let the choking begin...

The scene usually unfolds the same: The spoon approaches and food is hungrily taken in, only to be spewed out moments later. Yes, that's right. Mommy's dieting again. As for baby, she's just starting her unhealthy relationship with food. Sure, those sweet potatoes seem fairly innocent now, but when baby's busting out of size 6 Months, you'll have only Gerber and yourself to blame.

WHAT YOU MAY BE FREAKED OUT ABOUT
Once Bitten, Twice Bitten

"What are the signs that a tooth is on the way? There are gnaw marks on all her toys, but I don't see any tooth buds. Are squirrels to blame?"
Usually, but not in this case. Specifically, is baby pulling at his ear, rubbing his cheek, and in general being a pisser? If so, chances are you've got a little teether and will be seeing a tooth sprout in no time. Sometimes, the tooth fairy appears and the teeth come in painlessly and seemingly overnight. Other times, the tooth fairy is just not feeling the love (possibly from not meeting tooth quotas, and we won't even get into Santa inferiority complex) and in a fit of misdirected rage, decides to bitch-slap baby with her wand. Other teething signs:

Excessive saliva: baby looks like your husband in the presence of your college-aged sitter.

Facial irritation: a red ring around the mouth is a common side effect of constant drool. Why else do you think your husband grew that sad little goatee?

Biting: baby tears up everything in sight and, using See-and-Say Animals, tries to pin it on, naturally, squirrels.

Petting Zoo Precaution:

Innocent Sheep or Wool-Draped Terrorist?

There's nothing like a petting zoo to make baby's stuffed farm friends come to life right before her very eyes. What you may not see is the risk of E. coli that can be transferred from those innocent-looking cud-munchers. E. coli exposure can result in serious stomach ailments and can sometimes be deadly—talk about ruining a trip to the zoo. Other petting-zoo dangers? Goats and sheep alike find babies and their attire delicious. Turn your back for a moment and all that's left of your child is the clattering remains of the indigestible hardware from their OshKosh B'Gosh overalls. And that souvenir feeding-pellet necklace? Baaaa-d idea.

Unexpected Health Concerns

Lead: why kids keep getting dumber.

Everyone knows that lotsa' lead hurts the head. But even limited exposure can make your child sluggish, dim-witted, and a possible game-show participant. Household paint is one major source of lead, so be sure any painted products that your child comes in contact with are safe. Even a fresh coat of wall lacquer can hide a contaminated layer applied years before. Particularly, be cautious of painted antiques or imported toys. Most recently, toys manufactured in China have been cited as some of the most dangerous offenders. A few sips from that Hello Kitty tea set, and you'll have a baby who can see through walls—and possibly check for layers of lead!

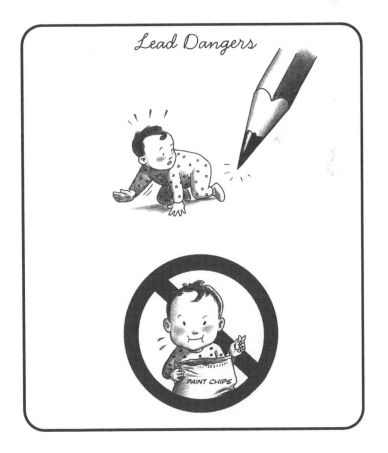

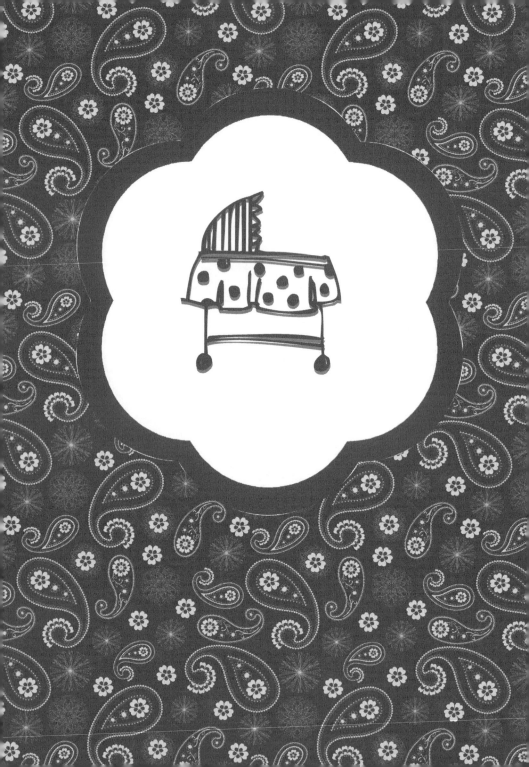

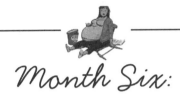

CHAPTER 17

Month Six:
Should Baby Be in
Preschool or Something?

Baby is like any social being now, smiling and cooing at every stranger they meet then ripping on them the moment they're out of earshot. At this point, baby's hands love to explore, especially your face. She will delight in pulling and twisting the sad remains of your thinning hair while teaching you that expensive sunglasses are virtually impossible to repair.

HOW FAR YOUR BABY LAGS BEHIND OTHERS
By Six Months, Baby...

...BETTER BE ABLE TO:

Keep head level or keep a level head even while you're relaying another embarrassing poop story about him.

...WILL MOST LIKELY BE ABLE TO:

Practice balancing on legs, just enough to realize you're the boss for now.

Fight your pets for anything that falls on the floor and is considered edible by infant/animal standards (i.e., anything that succumbs to gravity).

...MAY EVEN:
Say "mama" and "dada" at either parent, houseplants, or the refrigerator.

...WON'T BE ABLE TO:
Raise your credit score.

WELL-BABY CHECK: "AW, LOOK — SHE'S OLD ENOUGH TO KNOW TO BE AFRAID"

- Measurements: Assessment of baby's weight gain and silent assessment of yours.
- Developmental Check: Baby will be put through a series of tests, such as neck and head control and self-control when placed in front of a plate of delicious donuts. Other test include socialization ("Baby, who is on the cover of this week's *People*, what have they done lately, and why is it important? Because it is, you know.") and reflexes. ("Catch, baby! Well, you won't be going out for the Majors anytime soon.")
- Immunizations: Another round of baby-arm skewering— whoops, we mean shots.

BABY FOOD: STORE-BOUGHT OR MAKE YOUR OWN SALMONELLA...

Back when it was totally uncool to have children, you had to go about the unpleasant task of making/killing your own baby food. (That was, of course, when you weren't scrubbing the dung from cloth diapers or chopping the head off that night's dinner.) Now you can go to the store shelf and let a large faceless conglomerate do the prep work for you. As far as you're concerned, that tiny jar could contain pureed gizzard—just stick a bedimpled face on the label, hit fifteen seconds in the microwave, and you're the infant answer to Emeril. *Bam!* ("Whoops, sorry, baby.") But if parenting doesn't offer enough challenges, or you're just earthy and pretentious, you can still make your own baby food. (It's essential to tell everyone you have done so or the nutritional content is totally blown. That's just the rules.) You'll need to break out your blender. Not since your vibrator will you spend as much time with a loud, gyrating appliance, but it will be worth it for the sheer sense of superiority—oh, and that it's good for baby, blah, blah, blah...

WHAT YOU MAY BE FREAKED OUT ABOUT
Go Ahead and Make a Key for the Tooth Fairy

"My baby sprouted a chopper! Do I really need to start brushing it? Between brushing her hair and bathing the little rascal, I've got enough hygiene commitments."

Somewhere out there, a toothbrush is set aside and a hillbilly angel gets her wings...Baby teeth are going to fall out any way, you might reason (between smacks of Big Red gum, no doubt).

Don't wash away your concern with a swig of Mountain Dew just yet, Mom (or "sis," "aunt," "court-appointed guardian," or whatever inbreed family tree branch you've been assigned in baby's life). Your infant needs those early tooth nubs for biting and chewing. You need only look at the gnawed wood armrests of the alley-obtained futon in your living room as proof. Studies show a child who isn't introduced to good oral hygiene early in life has a higher risk of future tooth decay, speech impediments, and guest appearances on daytime talk shows.

Baby on Board:

Who's That Sleeping in My Bed? Everyone!

Don't feel like pushing a sleep-alone agenda? Or maybe you're looking for a legitimate out for perfunctory sex. Welcome to extended co-sleeping, which is slightly less weird than breastfeeding until they can obtain a learner's permit. The family bed can be a welcome haven for a mom and dad who don't have the time or funds to deal with marriage counseling. ("What if we wake the baby? Better not tonight...") Co-sleeping is part of the attachment-parenting philosophy, which subscribes to the notion that you are solely a vessel for all of your child's needs, there to be sucked dry, leaving a husk of your former self. Most important, both parents have to be on board the co-sleeping train. If not, prepare for a lot of out-of-town co-sleeping on the part of your partner.

Nighttime Crying: Will the Neighbors Hate Us Even More?

First it was the sounds of your arguments, occasionally followed by the clumsy sounds of lovemaking. Now it's your child's nighttime wailing that your neighbors must endure. *Where's a violent home invasion when you need one*, they sigh. It's understandable that neighborly relationships can easily be strained by a crying baby. Try not to be too self-conscious. Just think about how long you endured their yapping dog and how it took you *months* until you finally spiked that hamburger meat. Tolerance goes a long way. So does planting suspicion about the Joneses' troubled teenage son.

Here are some solutions to influence the folks next door:

"WON'T YOU BE MY NEIGHBOR" BOUNCER:
Borrow a slim, elderly gentleman from the local convalescent center. (Preferably one with no family to miss him.) Dress him in a cashmere sweater and post him at the door to deal with such matters. Who could be mad at a grandfatherly Mr. Rogers look-alike? Crisis averted.

NO SOUND AND SOME FURY:
Cover their house or apartment façade with soundproof, Styrofoam egg-crate material. If they can rip through it to get inside their home, it serves as a great noise insulator. Plus, everyone loves popping that stuff. Oh wait. That's bubble wrap. *Dammit!*

DISEASE DEFENSE:

Refer to some archaic medical condition ("Our little Billy is such a trooper in the face of scurvy!") and tell them it keeps baby up at all hours in pain. Then add conspiratorially, "But if he starts to disturb you, you come right to our door, and we'll see to it he's dealt with."

Bowel-Lingual

"My baby's bowel movements are totally schizophrenic—one day, odorless, hard, and a '70s brown, the next, pungent, runny and pea green." What are you? A diaper sommelier? This isn't a wine-tasting, subject to color and bouquet ("Complex, woody and round. Possible origin? Strained peas; vintage: lunchtime.") Take your face out of that cotton toilet and get a hold of yourself. Oh, and you've got something on your nose.

"THIS...SWING...ISN'T...GOING...TO... RAISE...ME."

By the six-month mark, your child has turned into a sophisticated little explorer. No longer is baby like malleable putty in your hands (unlike your husband in bed), and it will take more to entertain him than mirroring his awkward facial expressions (again, your husband in bed.) Here is what baby is working on and how you can help him develop beyond the limitations of an associate's degree.

The Big Stuff

These are the large motor skills necessary for sitting up, walking, and one day moving far, far away from you. Challenge baby to the tasks your pets never could seem to master, such as fetching the paper and actively liking you.

The Small Stuff

This is the finer motor coordination that will help your child feed himself, hold a crayon, open a bottle of pills, and possibly give a fantastic massage.

STUFFED TOYS:
Allow baby to act out the dramas occurring at home.

PHALANGE FUN:
Like itsy-bitsy spider, and point-the-blame…

HOW-TO PRETEND:
Offer baby a classic toy telephone but get ready for him to be mystified by this rare animal with a rotary dial. Babies also adore play cash registers, preparing them for a fallback career in retail.

Social Awareness

This age is a social gala for babies. They don't realize you should fear strangers, so their standards are relatively low when it comes to general fraternization. Introduce baby all over the place: to your friends, neighbors, and that hot guy who works out at your gym at 6 p.m. every Monday, Wednesday, and Friday and, during inclement weather, occasionally on Saturdays.

Language Acquisition

Baby is staring to comprehend. Words like "mommy" and "daddy" are becoming recognizable as are common phrases like "Ready to nurse?" and "That dog's butt is not a CD player." Other helpful tips for intellectual growth:

- Cause and effect games (Drop a ball—"See, it bounces back."—or tear up a credit card statement—"See, Daddy will never know").
- Explaining the sounds in his world. When a low-lying plane roars by, duck and scream, "Terrorists!" When a fire truck passes with its siren wailing, make note to baby, "I hope grandma didn't fall asleep smoking again." These experiences will also help with vocabulary building ("Grandma," "terrorist").
- Powers of observation. Point out: The blanket is fuzzy, the sun is warm, Mommy is numb.
- Let your child experiment. If your child is using toys in a nontraditional way ("Doctor, I don't know how Barbie's shoe got in there") try not to discourage her. When using household objects, explain what they are for: The mop is for cleaning the floor, the water is for washing dishes, this neck-massager isn't for necks at all.

Kudos! You made it through the first half of your baby's first year! By now, you're well on your way to a future filled with "I hate you!" and "Mom, I totaled the car—and failed math. Oh, and got a girl pregnant."

And when that time comes, you can hand him this book…

CHAPTER 18

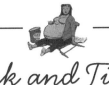

Sick and Tired
(The Baby, Not You)

Nothing is as upsetting as when your baby gets sick—except when baby gets you sick. Even if it's just the sniffles, an under-the-weather infant can upset any parent. This time, when vomiting occurs, you'll have to do more than hold someone's hair or clean the car later. You're solely responsible for getting your baby through their childhood ailments, and although they'll recover, that Jil Sander blouse may not.

FROM SNIFFLES TO SERIOUS PANIC
Hold the Phone

If baby is really sick, never hesitate to call the doctor. But a midnight call to the doc about a runny nose can make any physician reluctant to render aid. So weigh your concerns appropriately. Ask yourself: if *I* were the one who was ill, would it cause me to miss work? (Outside of big sales and drinking too much the night before.) If the answer is yes, then make the call. His alienated spouse probably didn't want to do it tonight, anyway.

Give Details

Don't assume your doctor has baby's chart memorized. Remind him of your child's age, medical history and distinguishing features. ("You remember my Janie...the really pretty one.") Mention possible exposures such as flu, a sibling with strep, or that witch's brew your mother-in-law calls food. Also have the number of your nearby pharmacy handy—and your seedy cousin's home lab doesn't count.

The 411 on Temperature

The doc's going to want to know. You've seen your mother and grandmother do it, but the old kiss-on-the-forehead, although comforting, is not accurate. (But more accurate than the elbow to the forehead.) Enter the thermometer.

Literally.

Taking the temperature at regular intervals can answer questions such as "Is the treatment working? and "Is it hot and crispy yet?" Oh. That's the oven timer. Hey, the pizza is ready!

PICK YOUR POISON

Say good-bye to that mercury thermometer—they're not endorsed any more due to chemical risk. (Specifically, the risk you'll want to break it and play with the neat, gray, shape-shifting liquid inside. To note, it's like the stuff that made up the evil cyborg in *Terminator 2: Judgment Day!* Awesome.)

Most often, the thermometer of choice is a digital thermometer. They're quite simple, really (especially if you can talk someone else into doing it for you). They can be used in the rectum, mouth or armpit. Basically, if you've got a hole, it's the thermometer for you. With a digital, you get a reading in less than a minute , which means everything when you're holding an infant down with only your forearm. Again, rely on visualization. Think of baby as the opposing lightweight contender and hold her to the mat (in this case, play mat). Remember, the title depends on it. Have your spouse act as referee, slapping the pinning surface for emphasis in those last crucial seconds. Three! Two! One!...*Beep*...*Beep*. Scale the nearest vista in victory climb. Oh, hold on a minute. You've got a sick kid on your hands. Save the dramatic celebration for when baby is well and can fully appreciate the level of his defeat.

REAR WINDOW

Relax before inserting the thermometer. You're going to have to put something in baby's behind so it's natural you'll need time to not be upset and grossed out. Try thinking of baby as an uncooked turkey. Add those tiny chef's hats as booties for maximum authenticity. Basting optional.

UNEXPECTED ENTRY: RECTAL INSERTION

Possibly from personal experience, you know there's nothing more disconcerting than when someone enters the backdoor without knocking. ("I don't care if it is your birthday. Consider it like the door at the movie theater—exit only.") When it comes to taking a temperature, baby is no less reluctant to Tango in Paris. You could offer the ol' "this hurts me just as much as it hurts you";

ironically, a phrase that could only be evenly delivered by someone *without* something in their anus. To make things easier, lubricate the tip thermometer first, then bare baby's bottom. If it helps, draw eyes and a nose on your baby's naked behind, allowing you to instead stare into the image of someone who, apparently, sucked too hard on a lemon or ingested alum. Aim the thermometer for the puckered "mouth" and—*voila!*—it will feel like an average oral temperature reading. Only to you, of course.

Other Symptoms to Note

BABY BEATS:

If baby's heart rate seems elevated and you haven't been leaping out and scaring him, make a note to your pediatrician.

BREATHING:

Note the rhythm. If it helps, place a light object on baby's chest to highlight the pattern like a small beverage. If it sloshes…damn, baby, what a mess!

WHEEZY BABY:

Is baby hacking? Does she sound like your older aunt who smokes clove cigarettes and hasn't ever mentioned a boyfriend? Another symptom to note…

GENERAL DEMEANOR:

Does nothing amuse baby? Even when you try to get into your pre-pregnancy jeans? If he can't even muster a snicker while observing you trying on swimwear, by all means, tell your doctor.

YOU, YOUR BABY'S PHARMACY

Sure, you know medication can be fun, but for baby, it's all business. (And possibly a profitable one in his teens and early twenties.) Here are the hard-and-fast rules for over-the-counter and prescription medication for infants.

- Don't use a drug if it has the word "tonic" anywhere on the label.
- If the directions of your medication conflict with your doctor's instructions, don't ask the pharmacist. If he knew better, he'd be a doctor. Instead, ask him where to find the frozen-food section or school-supply aisle. They love that.
- Never give baby your elderly father's medication. "Well, it's heart medicine—and coughing comes from near the heart." Cue ambulance siren.

Something's Going Down—Either the Medicine or You, Baby

Medicine is an unpleasant experience for most babies. One look at that dropper and baby will clamp up harder than you did when he took you to Chili's for your birthday. One method for getting your little guy to take his medicine is to demonstrate for him. Have your husband administer a few doses to you and gobble it greedily in front of baby. If you get dizzy or start to vomit, keep going. (Unless you want your child to be a quitter. A *sick* quitter.) If baby continues to battle, ask your doctor if you can get a higher concentration to allow for less dosing or try administering with a blow dart.

OTHER TAKE-IT-IN TIPS:

Approach baby with confidence. Half of winning the game is faking out your opponent. Before you bring his fever down, you have to bring baby down. Only when he's finally put in his place will the healing begin.

Distract baby with false sightings, such as "Hey, is that Big Bird in the laundry room?" or "Look! Elmo is in our breakfast nook!" As soon as he turns, give him that one-two grape punch.

Regale him with stories about "braver" and "better" babies who are taking their medication and getting well. It's never too early to set up an inferiority complex, requiring a different kind of medication in the future.

Allergy or Just Plain Ol' Intolerance?

If someone tells you that they are allergic to a certain food, that's an allergy. If someone tells you they're allergic to Hispanics, that's intolerance.

ALLERGIES

Loyal Household Friend or Four-Legged Allergen?

The general school of thought was that pets increase a child's chances of having allergies. But recent evidence suggests that a pet actually *reduces* your child's chance of becoming allergic. (Dog and cats in unison: "In your face, humans!") Does that mean if you have no pets, your doctor will be writing a script for one schnauzer, walk twice a day, dress and humiliate as needed? Hardly. Still, having baby slowly integrate with the already-present pets in your household is one way to maximize a breathing-friendly environment. For example:

- Have kitty sit near baby once a day, eventually progressing to a nuzzle, then licking his hand, to practically sitting on baby's face. (Just like it happened during your courtship!)

- Start a dialogue between baby and family dog. Explain to both how much they have in common: He loves to play with toys, you love to play with toys; he likes to slobber, you slobber; he was found in an alley…kidding, baby!

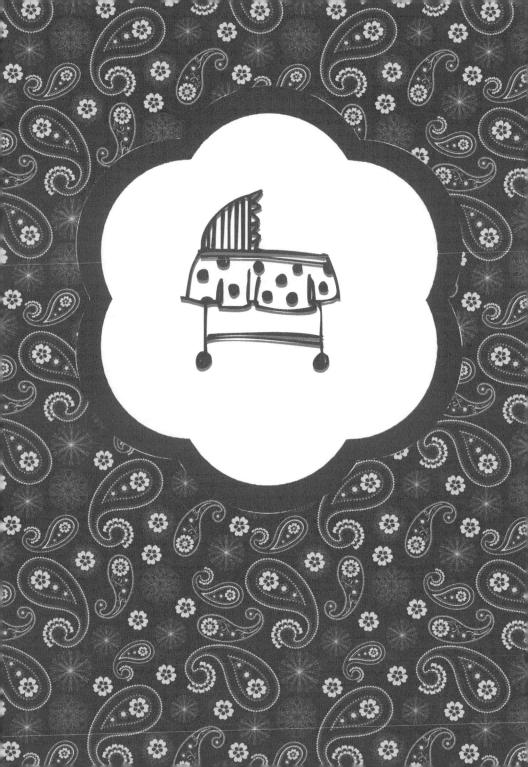

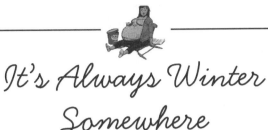

CHAPTER 19

It's Always Winter Somewhere

Female human beings can get pregnant any time of the year— especially the time of year they'd like to be engaged. But no matter when your baby is finally born, you'll be facing all types of elements in those initial twelve months. So whether baby is greeted by Christmas cheer or just a few months shy of that summer you'll be sitting out, you'll need to be prepared for any season under the sun...or snow.

WHAT YOU MAY BE FREAKED OUT ABOUT IN SUMMER WEATHER

Airing Baby Out

It's summertime. All baby needs is a diaper, right? Sure, if you air-dry your clothes, and your décor is inflatable. Not to say you should bundle your summer baby. For most infants, a single airy layer is sufficient. In fact, too much clothing can lead to heatstroke. (But you go ahead and layer this summer. Really. Layer.) Overall, your own comfort level is probably the best gauge for baby. Except if you're sweating when everyone is cold or you're shaking when most are comfortable. Then you may have to rely on others for a temperature check. Or get some antivenom—quick.

Whose Future is Bright Now?

What's the most important aspect of summer time care for infants?

Sunscreen.

Wrong.

Great-looking sunglasses. There's nothing that says more about your baby than the frames on his face. UVA and UVB protection are obvious plusses but don't let that override the style and brand. (No one *sees* protection from harmful rays. But everyone will notice an ill fit or an extra "N" in Chanel.) Whether he's sporting tiny Aviators or celeb-favored Dolce&Gabbana wraparounds, your baby will be well on his way to establishing a signature style. Notice how people point and gawk at him as you push him in his stroller. Wait! He's choking on his signature!

Small price to pay to be cool.

THE LOTION OF THE LAME: SUNSCREEN

After sunglasses and a bitchin' bikini or pair of cool trunks, you'll need to think about protecting baby from the sun. Remember, this isn't the skin-friendly sun of the '80s that with the aid of baby oil, sun reflectors, and Wham! turned your skin a warm, cocoa brown. (And still no ill effects except a few oddly shaped moles. Go figure!) Unlike then, today's sun is a relentless skin-searing bastard, feeding off the pink and the helpless. Infants have to be very careful of their thin skin, making them highly sensitive to both the sun's rays and constructive criticism.

RAY-BAN: RULES OF THUMB ABOUT THE SUN

- No amount of tanning is safe, but if you can't stand to look at baby's deathly pallor or are from L.A., you may want to try slathering him in sunless tanner. Bonus: you can sketch abs on baby's flabby mid-section, providing the tone and definition he sorely needs.
- Babies with fair skin and light eyes are most prone to sun damage, so they must be shielded at all times. Ethnic babies? Surf's up!
- The risk of sun damage is greatest between late morning and early afternoon. But you're inside watching your "stories" during those hours anyway.
- The reflection of snow on the ground can cause sunburn, so make sure baby is wearing sunscreen or a cover-up over her swimsuit. Hey, what month is this?
- If you live in a warm climate, baby will likely be exposed more than most, so always be armed with a large floppy hat or parasol. Ignore the shout-outs to Dr. Quinn, Medicine Woman.

Other Hot Weather Hazards

INSECT BITES

Most insects appear adorable with their oversized eyes and fluttering wings, but as any paranoid mom will tell you, almost all are deadly or at least can cripple you for life. (And in some cases, make you itch like crazy!) Keep baby out of areas where insects tend to congregate, such as near public garbage containers or that homeless person who hasn't moved since Tuesday.

LITTLE SWIMMERS

Swim classes are not recommended. At this point in his young life, your child can barely master tap water, much less a swimming pool. If you're still undeterred, just take a hard look at some of the swim instructors who spend their days marinating in the urine of local children. Do you really want the sun-baked paws of a failed gym teacher to be the sole barrier between your child and the pool drain? Plus, parents who enlist infants in such advanced classes tend to be the types who are slightly overinvested in their child's activities. You'll often find them clutching the chain link fence at the little league games screaming, "Jesus! The baseball is on a tee and you can't hit it?!? I have no son!" or, alternatively, dying of shame at a mall ("A *bunny* in overalls? *Hello!?* It's called a Build-A-*Bear* for a reason. Go back and do it right!"). So if you want to spend the next few years sitting in a carpool interrupted by "auditions" and hearing second-hand accounts of soul-crushing tirades, by all means, dive in.

WHAT YOU MAY BE FREAKED OUT ABOUT IN WINTER WEATHER
Bundle Up Your Bundle of Joy

It's wintertime. Snowflakes are falling and somewhere out there, according to the geniuses on Madison Avenue, a polar bear and a penguin share a soft drink. ("*Ahhhh!* Something to wash you down with! Refreshing!") In really extreme cold, mittens, socks, wool booties, scarf, long-sleeve T-shirt, hat, sweater, insulated pants, and bunting suit should all be used for outdoor exposure. In the end, if you can safely bounce your child down a flight of stairs; or if she looks like the illegitimate child of the Michelin Man, consider yourself prepared.

What are some other ways to keep Jack Frost from nipping at your child's nose? (As long as Jack Frost doesn't live across the street and have a blue square over his house on the map of your neighborhood.) Here are some tips to keep baby warm and safe when Old Man Winter approaches. (Again, if you have any suspicions, check with local authorities.)

- Babies enjoy warming up by the fire just as much as adults do. But obviously, precautions must be taken. Make sure baby never sits too close or is left unattended. For more even warmth, slip a cool andiron down baby's coat and spin rotisserie style.

- Don't worry about baby becoming sick if he's temporarily exposed to cold. Colds are caused by viruses, not weather. Old people will argue with you all day about this. (Literally. Besides getting the mail, they have the entire day to do so.) Luckily, fragile bones and ice are a much more perilous combination. Old Mrs. Johnson won't feel so superior when she's flat on her back like a turtle. But remember, this is no time to begrudge a well-meaning advisor. Be sure to honk and wave.

MERRY MISHAPS: BEDECK AND BEWARE

'Tis the season…for lacerations? Certainly no baby has stitches on his Christmas wish list. But hidden in the holly and electrical trees are countless dangers that can potentially mar baby. (Not to be confused with "myrrh.") Whether it's pointy menorahs, the choking hazard of the tiny baby Jesus, or just the proliferation of mischief-making elves, baby has to watch his stocking-footed step lest he end up in the ho-ho-hospital. ("So little Billy, wheel on over here and tell me what you want for Christmas!") Here are some seasonal precautions:

MISTLETOE:
It's poisonous when eaten, not to mention baby will be forced to kiss people nearly forty times his own age.

HOLLY:
Only poisonous in large amounts, so baby can tolerate in moderation. Same goes for annoying cousin of the same name.

ANGEL HAIR:
Avoid altogether. This spun glass is sort of like decking the halls with raw insulation.

SNOW GLOBES:
They can be breakable and possibly give baby a God-complex about being able to control the weather.

EVERGREEN:
Real evergreen is a fire hazard, while the Barbra Streisand duet version will make you wish for a fiery death.

ALCOHOL:

It only takes a moment for baby to down an unattended cocktail and end up with alcohol poisoning. Although it can be a temporary scare for any parent, admit it: there's a part of you that totally understands.

ARRIVING ALIVE: THE HOLIDAY HOW-TO
Flying

Remember when you looked forward to vacations? This was before your diaper bag was a suspected explosive. Millions of people will fly during the holiday season, and if you're traveling with an infant or toddler, half of those people will hate you and your kind. (The other half will be carrying a carseat.) With that suspect stroller and bottles of breast milk that could go off at any moment, you're one big domestic hiccup at security check. Thanks to new airport security measures, you get to enjoy the delightful overlap between packing to meet Grandma and packing to meet Allah. ("Innocent teddy bear? We'll see about that." *Riiii-ipppppp!*) But that crack airport security team is only doing its job. Besides, how many more terrorists with their mom bobs and sensible Keds must slip through undetected before someone takes action?

So, how can you discern the fine line between mom and terrorist? Try to match the below phrases with the correct desperate and controlling tyrant.

- "I swear to God, I will turn this thing around!"
- "Everyone down on the ground—and pick up that mess!"
- "Don't make me come back there!"

- "Answer me!"
- "I'll give you something to cry about!"
- "I'm going to give you to the count of three…"
- "Over my dead body!"

See, it's not as easy as you think.

OTHER IN-FLIGHT INSTRUCTIONS

- Arrive in time to wrangle the kids and navigate security. Essentially, arrive the week before.
- Make sure to feed baby during the plane's take off and landing. Especially breast-feeding. It will help with baby's ear pressure and you'll avoid stares from the looming perv headed to the bathroom for the fifteenth time.
- If your baby cries uncontrollably, ask him to fill out a form instead.
- Pack a variety of small activities to keep baby engaged. But if your child does act up en route by crying and spilling things, ignore glares from flight attendants or other passengers. Simply make loud comments about the trip to get baby a new liver/heart/kidney and let the chips fall where they may (or pretzels, peanuts, trail mix…)

Throw Mama from the Train…

The train's whistle isn't the only thing that blows. If you're traveling by train domestically, you're in for a tunnel full of disappointment. Hardly the glamour coaches depicted in movies, your cut-rate ride will likely be one step up from a hobo car—and at least those allow you to hop on and off as needed. Imagine a budget hotel on wheels with an even more frugal passenger base. Not to mention, the general age of the conductor and fellow passengers will make you believe you just stepped on a shuttle to meet St. Peter. Here are some tips on surviving the *Disorient Express:*

- Arrive early to get the first seat of the car. If a disabled passenger in a wheelchair arrives there first, just unlock his brake and let the train's momentum do the dirty work for you.
- Scenery is as good as any toy: trees, animals in pastures, rows of houses, the couple making out in front of you...
- Keep children safely seated by telling them you think the train won't run out of track.

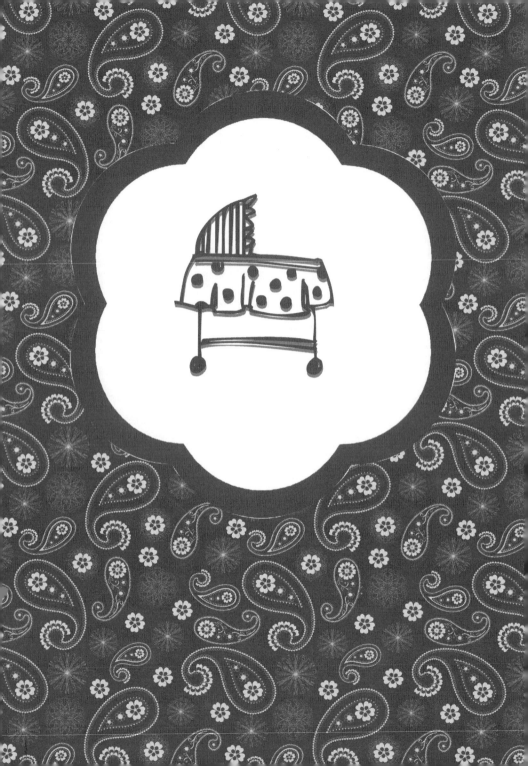

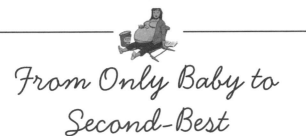

CHAPTER 20

From Only Baby to Second-Best

As second-time-around parents, you're practically experts. You can diaper a baby while you sleep (which explains baby waking up looking like a disheveled Sikh) and aren't daunted when an umbilical cord stump falls into your coffee ("Mmm! Navel-y!"). This time, it will be your firstborn who's in the hot seat. (Yeah. That kid who keeps hanging around and asking for food.) There will be some bumps ahead, but try not to worry. You need only to make sure your first baby understands that you have enough love for everyone. Here are a couple of do's and don'ts for an expanding family.

Do: Have them spend the night at Grandma's for a little independence.
Don't: Cruise orphanages and ask elder child, "So what do you think?"

Do: Let your child help prepare the baby's nursery.
Don't: Offer your child the want ads, with the real-estate section highlighted.

WHAT YOU MAY BE FREAKED OUT ABOUT
Been There, Done That—"That" Is You

"We have a three-year-old, and we're trying for a cuter baby. How can we introduce the idea to our firstborn in a way he'll understand?"

Thanks to those kids and their Internet, you can't exactly tell your ten-year-old Timmy the stork impregnated you. Today, sibling instruction is of the utmost importance to help ensure a successful family transition. Your first child will want to be included, but it's important to do so in a way he can comprehend. This isn't the time to tell your kid about your tilted cervix or the inherent risks of placenta previa. Break the news honestly and in simple language: *We're going to have a baby. Mommy is happy, but Daddy is having mixed feelings. Oh, don't worry. He loves you—now that you have a personality and all. It's just baby is inside Mommy's tummy and doesn't quite seem real. At least not real to the jerk who doesn't have to endure the morning sickness and unbearable fatigue. Anyway, in case you were silently accusing me of getting fat, I just want to make things clear: I'm pregnant. So you can stop looking at me that way when I order my mochachino with whip. The good news is, you're going to have a little sister or brother. The bad news is, you're going to have to split our assets with someone else one day. Congratulations! Now move out of your room. There's a new kid in town.*

OTHER TIPS FOR EASING INTO FULL-BLOWN SIBLING RIVALRY:

- Highlight all the advantages of being an older sibling. Remind your child of both the physical and mental intimidation edge that can be lorded over baby now and for years to come. For example, when they're children, she'll have better, more advanced toys than little sis; in her teens, she'll have better, more advanced breasts—making getting all the boys' attention a cinch.

- Don't bring up sibling issues unless your child does first. Don't say, "Don't worry. I bet this baby won't be more attractive than you"; or "It's really doubtful you'll need to get a job to help with finances."

- Have her "meet" the baby while you're still pregnant. Show your firstborn monthly fetal development through ultrasound printouts or have them yell a greeting up your skirt.

- Take your child to your check-up appointments. She'll feel like a part of the process and get to hear firsthand about the baby from your doctor. To avoid awkwardness during physical exam, simply explain the doctor lost his keys and has to look everywhere to find them.

- Involve your child in sorting her old things for baby's use. You can also use this opportunity to get rid of non-essentials from babyhood like broken toys and tattered stuffed animals. Expect your firstborn to have mixed feelings. For you, it will feel like mass spring cleaning; for her, a mass execution of all her beloved childhood companions. Try to ease the loss with a reasonable explanation: sometimes we run out of room and our little friends are sent away to live in lesser homes. A perfect cautionary tale for sibling's arrival!

- If your first born uses the middle seat, move her car seat to a side seat. Fasten a doll in infant seat beside hers. She can practice expressing their mutual hate of Celine Dion.

- Let him be part of naming the baby. Keep in mind that older names like Elmo and Grover are making a huge comeback.

- Explain your body's changes but don't blame the baby. Instead, point to Daddy saying, "I can't get into it in detail, but bring all of your complaints up with that guy."

"I Don't Know How Baby Fell on Her Head—I Swear"

"There's already tension between our firstborn and newborn. I'm almost certain I overheard my oldest conspiring with our jealous dog to overthrow this 'new regime.' How can we ease the tension?"

Most parents are tempted to admonish such candor, but it's good for your child to express her frustrations. The best solution is to empathize with your child. Instead of telling her that it's bad for her to feel negatively toward this new intruder, go along with it and throw in some complaints of your own:

- "Babies are so lame. They can't even hold their heads up."
- "He poops his pants. I mean, *all* the time."
- "I'm not going to lie. I've seen prettier."
- "What's up with her fascination with *Baby Einstein?* I could shoot that in my living room with a music box, some wooden toys, and a felt backdrop."

"No, He Doesn't Have a Tail in the Front"

"Our four year old daughter wants to know everything about her baby brother's penis—things like how will it help catapult him up the corporate ladder. How should we address this?"

In simple language. Tell her girls have vaginas so they can have babies. Men have penises so they have access to vaginas. The fact is, children are often as fascinated by penises as they are eyes or noses. Treat her interests as benignly as you would any inquiry. And if she still won't relent, tell her that hers fell off from asking too many damn questions.

How to Raise a Hater

"I was worried about our five-year-old daughter being envious of the baby—but nothing! How do I shake her up to be slightly insecure, but not inconvenient-eating-disorder insecure?"

Sibling rivalry is normal, but not all children experience it. But if you want to stoke the flames of jealousy, just to ensure everybody loves Mommy, here are some tried-and-true methods guaranteed to turn your household into a Greek tragedy.

- Have "who's more adorable" auditions each evening. Feel free to include categories such as talent, congeniality, and swimwear. Winner gets to sleep in Mommy's bed.
- When your firstborn draws a picture, place it on the fridge then ask your infant, "So where is yours?" After you and eldest share a laugh about it, narrow your eyes, remarking, "You know, your giggle was a lot cuter as a baby."
- When your older child isn't looking, take a ragged saw to her Barbie's feet then complain loudly about baby's teething habits. Let the drama naturally unfold later at Barbie's condo.

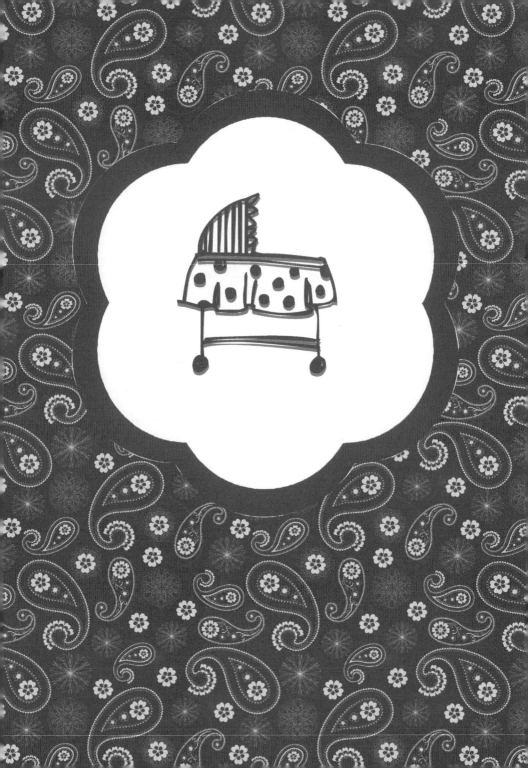

CHAPTER 21

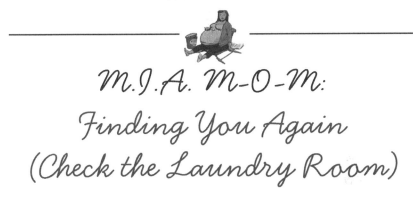

M.I.A. M-O-M:
Finding You Again
(Check the Laundry Room)

Yes, you're a mom now, but remember that person that used to dress well and have a great body? Okay, so you'll never be like your childless friend from college. But you can avoid the pitfalls of the becoming a mompod. Here's how to avoid getting caught in the tracksuit trap.

NEW MOM MISSTEPS:
Bad Clothes: The New Birth control

Somewhere along the way of wearing elastic maternity pants, some mothers begin to blur the boundaries when it comes to appropriate day wear. During pregnancy, it may have been okay to wear roomy pajamas and overalls* but if you ever want daddy to open the flap (also not unlike on the farm!) avoid these new-mom no- nos.

---

*It was never okay.

- Wearing something from a designer you've met—at your cousin's baby shower.
- Buying clothing emblazoned with a sentiment or flag; worse, a sentiment and a flag.
- Florals: It's all bad—no exceptions.
- Anything sold as a set or off television.
- Clothing designed by a television personality.
- Fashions purchased in the same place you can buy dry goods or souvenirs.

A good litmus test: If fellow moms gush that your clam diggers are "so cute" or go crazy over your denim jumper, clearly you're not fashion forward. If you are left off the PTA email list or treated like suspected terrorist at Gymboree, consider yourself a fashion success!

WHAT YOU MAY BE FREAKED OUT ABOUT
Work it, Part II

"I want to get back in shape, but you try affording a sitter for regular workouts. And then there's that whole thing about them wanting you to move around and all."

Who says you have to leave baby out of the act of getting fit? There are groups of new moms dedicated to getting in shape with baby in tow. You've seen them in park. They're the sidewalk bullies getting their cardio pushing a stroller at leisurely pace or breaking a sweat with two-pound barbells. These fitness groups usually have clever names like Buff-with-Baby or Fit2BeMamas, and meet a maximum of once a week so long as the weather is great, no one's husband is off, and it doesn't interrupt anyone's book club meeting. When they're not in the park, you can find them gathered at the local Olive Garden, filling up on free salad and heroic amounts of breadsticks. If you want to shed the baby weight just in time for your child's college graduation, by all means, this is the fitness club for you.

Or you can get a *temporary* eating disorder like a normal person and see real results. The key is temporary! Depending on your choice of weight purge, you can join the laxative crowd (Flush&Fit!) or the bulimic branch (Hur12BeHot!) Other people opt for the diet-pill route which, although effective, can kill you if mixed with a double espresso. Of course, some people take it too far, but you've seen way too many cautionary tales on E! to ever let that happen. Besides, even if you do die, you'll eventually reach your goal weight—just not in the way you expected.

Sexual Healing

"My doctor says it's okay to have sex. Do we have to?"
Don't be alarmed by lack of sexual desire. Keep in mind, it was only weeks ago your husband saw your vagina literally looking back at him. And in your case, you've had something inside of you for nine months, so you're kind of over it. There are other ways to express your love that don't involve coitus, including massage, hand-holding, and spying on your neighbors as *they* have sex. Another aspect is to cultivate your emotional versus physical connection until the sparks start to fly on their own. Here are some tips:

- Pick an annoying acquaintance, relative, or child and despise them together. A fault-finding mission can be as cohesive as any romantic getaway.

- Combine your individual perfect days. Don't worry about the second looks you'll receive while sharing a pedicure at Home Depot. Leaf-blow-dry, then relax in the outdoor swing section. Having keys made to each other's hearts optional.
- For the more adventurous, try mutual masturbation. Occasionally, yell over to your spouse in the other room and tell them how it's going.

Still Strung out...

"My baby is six months, and I'm still wiped out! Isn't there some college out there with an early-admissions program for this kid?"

Exhaustion can be caused by lots of things: an irregular schedule, lack of exercise, or just being a lazy bitch. But we all know caring for a newborn can be as emotionally draining and physically depleting as any job—even celebrity dog stylist. That's why it's important to not be too hard on yourself. (That's for society and your infertile friends to do for you.) So what if Baby Tylenol is your go-to liquid lullaby. Speak up, all you parents who have let the dog occasionally monitor the baby! (*Sound of crickets.*) Ironically, motherhood is not for pussies. All of these factors in mind, it's important not to rule out physical causes of fatigue. Remember, you are still in the postpartum triathlon that is the first year. Along with numerous lifestyle changes, your body is likely still accommodating to the hormonal whirlwind that is just winding down. Your breasts may still be tender, your period delayed...

Then again, you could be pregnant.

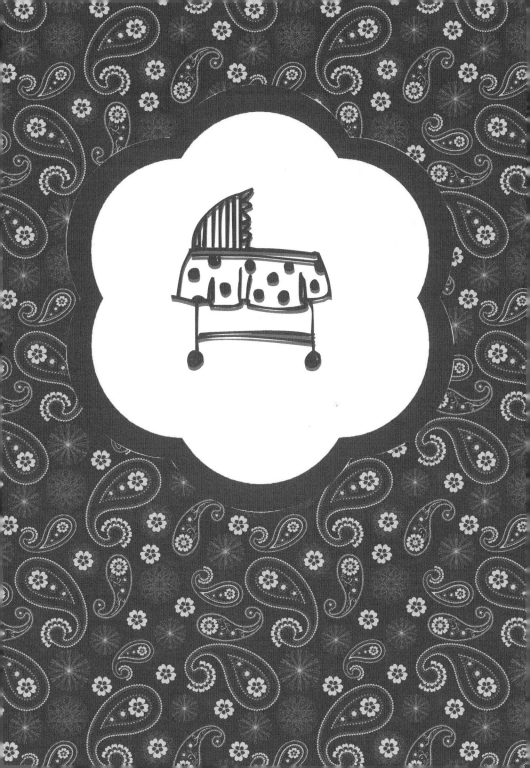

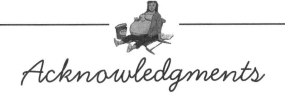

Acknowledgments

My sincerest thanks to Patty Curtis, friend and reader, who makes New York as close as my inbox. Also, enormous gratitude to my advocate and agent Barbara Zitwer who knows when to say " I love it!" or "It's dead, kid. What's next?" I'm also grateful to have fallen into the skilled editorial hands of Shana Drehs, whose hilarious and encouraging manuscript notes had me giggling at 3 a.m. (the hour when both mothers and the undead get most of their work done.) Other deserving nods: my legal eagles Keith Stanley, Danielle Claudat, and Ragan Melton, and various other superheroes who saved the day. And to John, who makes me laugh.

Closer to home, thank you to my solid little sleeper, S.K., whose straw-colored hair was often entwined in my left hand as my right was typing. Finally, to my husband, T.J., who during those uncertain days in New York in September 2001, gave me a certainty I didn't know possible—by asking me to marry him. *Unexpected*, indeed.

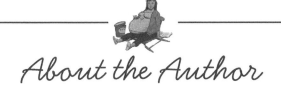

About the Author

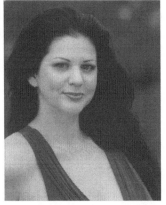

© Brenda Ladd

For ten years, Mary K. Moore worked as an editor and writer for a variety of New York publications including *Cosmopolitan*, *Redbook*, and *Marie Claire*. She's also written for *Glamour*, *Self*, *Newsweek*, and *Texas Monthly*, among others, with a focus on news features and essays. She's appeared on *Inside Edition*, *New York One*, *Extra*, *Access Hollywood*, and *Good Day New York*, speaking on topics ranging from parenting and relationship advice to celebrity news. She lives in Austin, Texas, with her husband, T.J., and their three-year-old daughter, Scarlett, and is secretly in love with motherhood.